GUIDED EMPATHY MERIDIAN TAPPING

GUIDED EMPATHY MERIDIAN TAPPING

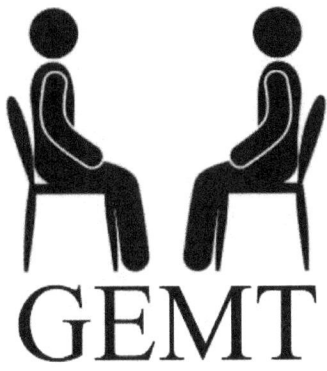

GEMT

GEMT® Practitioner Certification Manual

A Guide to Facilitate the Healing of "Victim Disease"

Robert Ranche and Dorthy Tyo

This book is presented to provide education, information and motivation and is not intended as a substitute for medical or psychological advice from the medical community. The reader should consult a physician in matters relating to health and symptoms that may require diagnosis or medical attention. The authors and the publisher are not engaged to render any type of professional medical advice. We are aware that there are other modalities available for study and practice for practitioners, professional or not, and our intention is to add to your choices for eliciting wellness in the lives of clients, patients, and of course, yourself. While best efforts have been used in preparing this book, the author and publisher make no representations or warranties of any kind and assume no liabilities of any kind with respect to the accuracy or completeness of the contents and specifically disclaim any implied warranties. Reading this book does not constitute a client-practitioner relationship between the reader and authors. Any and all others related to this publication do not assume any responsibility for how the reader chooses to apply information and techniques. As in all things, you are responsible for your own choices, actions and results.

Note: In case studies and instructions, we are utilizing female pronouns as a conscious choice to re-balance the historic gender imbalances of the English language.

Robert Ranche and Dorthy Tyo
Visit our website at www.GEMT.me

First Printing: March 2021

ISBN: 9798719158785

GEMT is a registered trademark of Robert Ranche and Dorthy Tyo

GRATITUDE

This book could not have happened without the help of many. A huge thanks to our amazing editors Lori Krein and Susan Dobra for their conscientious examination and quest for reader clarity. A big thank you to our fantastic reviewers: Lata Ramesh, Jan Allegretti, Dylan Rumley, John Marshall and Dina Zuccaro for organizing the flow of the material and to Lisa Petrocchi for all of her cheerleading. Dorthy specifically thanks Carol Simone and Susanna Juarez for their wisdom, suggestions and inspiration. Bob specifically thanks Catherine Carey for her love and support, Rosemeire Ranche for her spiritual wisdom, and Athena Demetrios for her inspiration, motivation and belief in this project. We both sincerely thank the hundreds of enthusiastic GEMT students at the Palo Alto School of Hypnotherapy.

Table of Contents

Introduction

"Man's mind, once stretched by a new idea, never regains its original dimensions." — Oliver Wendell Holmes

We wrote this book because we discovered a miraculous phenomenon everyone should know about. We, as humans, are born with a type of *infantile amnesia*, which, metaphysically speaking, includes a forgetting of any decision-making processes prior to birth. This anomaly creates plenty of opportunity to develop the belief in victimhood causing negative emotions to be held in the body and subconscious, thereby manifesting dis-ease, and contributing to negative behaviors. However, we have developed a process for overturning the subconscious belief of victimhood and have been teaching it since 2012. We share this with you because we believe this level of re-empowerment and healing belongs to all of us.

It is time for us, as a society, to change the way we look at chronic disease. We tend not to question the pain from touching a hot stove or an ulcer induced by stress, though many with chronic illnesses perceive themselves as victims of a malfunctioning body. They fixate on relief, hand-over their healing authority, and defend their belief in being powerless, which impedes their understanding that negative emotions cause dis-ease. Yet, when victimhood is replaced by self-responsibility, holistic health is restored.

In addition, victimhood and disempowerment are synonymous and the basis for all unrest. A deep seeded belief in victimhood creates a perception of limited choices and powerlessness other than the ability to commit crimes and acts of aggression. Many identify with victimhood, seeing it as part of who they are, self-perpetuating a perception of weakness, inability to respond, and lack of accountability. However, when we perceive ourselves as creators rather than victims of these difficult situations, a sense of ease, empowerment and freedom are restored.

We don't like to think of ourselves as victims even when we perceive things are happening *to* us rather than *for* us. People suffer when they believe they are victims, and throughout this book we refer to this belief as "Victim Disease." Whether from illness, abuse or other harm, the core of this suffering comes from the belief we did not choose the harmful situation. However, we do not believe we are a victim when we perceive our choices had something to do with its creation. Victimhood can be replaced by taking responsibility for any situation we believe we have created, and common logic tells us we must have something to do with every situation we are a part of, based on our choices and participation.

Though we often perceive ourselves as victims of harmful situations, we certainly take partial, if not all, credit as the creator of favorable situations and outcomes. We either accept that we are at least part creator of all situations, whether good or bad, or not a creator of anything. When we take credit for the difficult situations as we do the favorable ones, we begin to understand ourselves as true creators. There is an experience of exaltation when we realize we have the ability to respond, from deep within us, as the creator of our life experiences. This acknowledgement of self-responsibility has been recognized to heal and is the basis of GEMT. Much of this book is focused on the philosophy of how to be at ease with clients and their issues so that this transformation can take place. We have found, through our studies and years of practice, that shifting our perception from being a victim to that of a creator transforms subconscious beliefs and allows deep healing to happen.

Some healing modalities find value of traumatic events so the client can "own" them. However, the difference between owning and choosing is enormous. Suggesting clients feel better about something they believe they did not choose can deepen victimhood and disempower future choices. Other healing modalities fabricate comforting memories yet maintain victimhood and unworthiness. GEMT does not fix nor see emotions from traumatic events as the issue, but the perception it was not chosen. GEMT focuses on the client seeing herself as the creator of her difficult situations, choosing to experience specific traumatic events for valuable purposes.

We are profoundly aware that the idea of being a creator rather than a victim may be nearly impossible for some people to entertain or embrace. For many, the thought of looking at their most victimized experience can be as painful as surgery without anesthesia. However, just as the discovery of general anesthesia transformed medicine, the recent discoveries of what we call "Emotional Anesthesia" have transformed aspects of cognitive therapy. There are two other popular emotional anesthesia techniques, 1. bilateral stimulation and 2. breathing with muscle relaxation. However, meridian tapping was the breakthrough discovery for us. Not only can meridian tapping be done in a way that incorporates bilateral stimulation, it also provides for mirroring/matching which helps create an empathetic rapport. This rapport helps the practitioner guide the client to a plausible and beneficial explanation of a traumatic event. GEMT (pronounced: gem-tee) essentially guides the client back to the time when she gave up her power so that she can reclaim it. This level of healing would be nearly impossible without both emotional anesthesia and empathetic rapport, and the reason why meridian tapping is in the name of this modality. Thanks to these recent discoveries, the discomfort of healing can be minimized.

When we began helping clients change their perception from victim to that of creator, we discovered an extraordinary level of healing that is far beyond what we had set out to accomplish. We are not saying that this is the only way but are very sure that GEMT is a reliable, empowering, restorative modality. GEMT is designed to help you help others in transforming their old perceptions and beliefs that have impeded their life's journey and obstructed their dreams, goals, purposes, and birthrights.

In the process of teaching this modality, we have introduced terms to aid in the understanding of the concepts. "Subconscious Veto," "Subconscious Guilt," "Emotional Anesthesia" and "Victim Disease" are terms we found in no other modalities at the time, and we utilize them to help the student gain better clarity for this new approach to healing. They are not meant to be defined or redefined beyond the scope of this book.

It's true. We see ourselves as healers and we believe everyone is a healer at some level. The mother who kisses a scraped elbow to "make it better," the man who puts his arm around a despondent friend and tells him "better days are ahead," the minister/priest who absolves sins, the friend or stranger who just sits and listens; it's all about healing in one way or another. We are inspired by your willingness to explore the boundless possibilities of this unique modality and embrace the adventure of healing the illusion of victimhood...from *victim* to *victorious*!

Robert Ranche and Dorthy Tyo

Building Blocks for Learning GEMT

Start at level 1 on the bottom. Each level builds on the previous one below it.

─────────────── **LEVEL 9 - Self-responsibility as The Creator** ───────────────

| Offer the Pivotal "Why Would I Create This?" | Present Value for Choosing the Core Issue Situation | Client Thanks Ailment/Discomfort/People for Helping Realize she is The Creator |

─────────────── **LEVEL 8 - Find the Core Victimhood Issue** ───────────────

| Define the Emotional Element of the Dis-ease | The Emotion Corresponds to an Early Childhood Response | Client Recognizes the Victimhood Perspective was Learned in Early Childhood |

─────────────── **LEVEL 7 - The Healing Approach** ───────────────

| When to Use GEMT | Only Work on What the Client is Ready to Work on | Help the Client Be at Ease with her Ailment and Situation | Relief is not Healing / Ailments have Value |

─────────────── **LEVEL 6 - How to Be for the Client** ───────────────

| Be at Ease / Nothing is Wrong | Perceive the Client Is Right Where She Should Be | Recognize Valuable Healing Opportunities | Perceive the Client as Part of Yourself |

─────────────── **LEVEL 5 - Healing Perspective** ───────────────

| How and Why to Be Empathetic / The Emotion is Never Wrong for the Perspective | How and Why to Be Non-Judgmental / The Past is Unchangeable, Do No Harm, All Ailments Have Value |

─────────────── **LEVEL 4 - Tools for Healing** ───────────────

| Higher the Vibration Clearer the Perspective | Desensitization Prerequisite for Confronting Painful Memories | Rapport is Key to Guiding the Client | Influence Healing with the Power of Empathy |

─────────────── **LEVEL 3 - Healing Measurements** ───────────────

| The Vibration Scale of Emotions | Subjective Units of Discomfort Scale (SUDS) | Quantifying Success Affirms to the Subconscious that Healing has Occurred |

─────────────── **LEVEL 2 - Understanding Disease** ───────────────

| Misbeliefs Create Dis-ease | Emotional Reactions are Learned | Victimhood is a Perception "Victim Disease" | GEMT Only Focuses on Victim Disease |

─────────────── **LEVEL 1 - Fundamental Elements** ───────────────

| What is GEMT? Overturns Victimhood with Self-Responsibility so the Client can Heal Herself | What is Dis-ease? Negative Emotions from Misperceptions Cause Dis-ease | What is Healing? A Shift in Perception from Suffering Toward Wholeness | What is Healer? A Healer Facilitates Healing / We are all Healers |

PART 1 – What is GEMT?

"A vivid imagination compels the body to obey it..." – Aristotle

What is GEMT?

Guided Empathy Meridian Tapping (GEMT) is a holistic adventure and a therapeutic intervention for replacing victimhood with self-responsibility. This heals what we call "Victim Disease." It does this by first bringing ease to what has manifested, not to fix, modify, neutralize, mask, or remove any issue. When there is ease about the ailment, the cause is readily found as the misperception of victimhood developed early in life. GEMT sees that the traumatic event is not the issue, it's the dis-ease from perceiving it as not chosen. The ultimate goal of GEMT is to facilitate the client's understanding that she is not a victim and is responsible for manifesting her ailment so that she can choose to heal it.

Scientific Hypothesis

We have yet to prove in scientific terms how the GEMT method of healing works. However, by researching similar physiological conditions and effects, we believe our logical explanations can be used as a reasonable theory. Many of the terms are explained in later chapters.

1. Prior to the client choosing her issue and establishing a beginning *Subjective Units of Distress Scale* (SUDS) level, she feels a sense of safety, clarity and higher cognitive functions by experiencing *heart coherence* from positive emotions.

2. The client's chosen issue is viewed as a result of *classical conditioning* originating at an event prior to the age of eight.

3. The *emotional anesthesia* from the *bilateral stimulation* of *acupressure points* allows the client to confront the event with minimal discomfort.

13

4. As the practitioner empathetically offers a plausible beneficial explanation of why she might choose to create such an event, her *mirror neurons* provide her the experience of being the creator.

5. Perceiving herself as the creator instead of the victim, her body regains stress-resilience by the release and rebalancing of the neurochemical *neuropeptide Y* (NPY).

6. The difference in *SUDS* level at the end of the session confirms to her *subconscious* that healing has happened.

The GEMT Method

When you see "tapping," you might think GEMT is similar to other tapping modalities such as Thought Field Therapy (TFT) or Emotional Freedom Techniques (EFT). However, because of GEMT's unique approach to healing, we ask you to set aside any knowledge you might have of other tapping modalities, other than the tapping points, while learning GEMT. GEMT is not similar to other tapping modalities because it does not focus on fixing, modifying, or removing symptoms, seeing them as an effect, not a cause. GEMT views dis-ease as overreactions to a perceived separation from oneness and cherishes these overreactions because they are key to overturning the perception victimhood.

Whether physical or emotional, GEMT treats all ailments as emotional dis-ease and views physical issues as negative emotions stored in the body. All physical diseases and discomforts have an emotional element. When working with a physical issue it is first converted to an emotion, so that the core emotional event can be found. When working with emotional issues we typically can jump straight to the core issue. *GEMT treats all ailments as emotional dis-ease.*

Meridian tapping itself does not do the healing, but it provides what we call a temporary "emotional anesthesia" which reduces negative emotions and defensiveness about the ailment, so that practitioners can empathetically guide clients to a perspective that their ailment has value. The suggested value is that the ailment is an indicator of a much bigger issue buried in the client's subconscious that has similar emotions. Once guided back to the earlier issue, the practitioner intuitively offers her a plausible beneficial explanation for why the distressing situation occurred, helping her take responsibility for it. The client gains the understanding that she can choose to heal her ailment once she accepts responsibility for it. This understanding produces an internal shift that often has profound life-changing effects.

The four components of a GEMT session are:

- The practitioner has enough empathetic influence to guide the client.
- The client has a lower defensiveness when tapping on meridian points.
- The client physically and verbally participates in the healing process.
- The practitioner is able to guide the client to perceive value for her difficult situation.

One of the unique qualities that makes GEMT different from other modalities is that it does not focus on healing the dis-ease; it focuses on healing the reaction to the dis-ease, and when the reaction is healed (understood, transformed, transmuted) there no longer seems to be a need or use for the dis-ease. A negative reaction can be interpreted as a response learned while experiencing a feeling of victimhood. The GEMT perspective is to view a current negative reaction as a valuable opportunity to change misperceptions developed earlier in life.

Based on the theory that every current action is based on a previous action; we offer the idea that a change in our interpretation of a past action will have a ripple effect on interpreting subsequent actions. Wanting or wishing for a different past is essentially being in discord with all that is now. We feel there is no greater dis-ease than to be in resistance to the past, which is unchangeable. GEMT focuses on finding value for a past event and accepting it. This creates an ease that can only come from accepting the past.

Beneficial Side Effects

Clients have reported profound life-changing effects as a result of a GEMT session. We cannot ignore the comments of the many GEMT clients who claim that overcoming their dis-ease was one of their most important accomplishments. Great and rapid explicit and implicit learning has occurred in these clients through the understanding that their suffering is a result of their own choices. Clients have reported improved relationships, life balance, abundance, success and overall well-being. The most valuable side effect of GEMT is the client's realization that they are responsible for ALL of their life experiences.

Some of the reported beneficial *realization* side effects are:
- Everything has value, and suffering and dis-ease are no exception.
- A situation has a purpose regardless of whether it is perceived as good or bad.
- At certain times we all innocently play healing roles for each other.
- Judging and condemning is unhealthy for everyone.
- We all have the power to heal ourselves.
- We are much more powerful than we believe we are.
- We can reclaim our power to love unconditionally.

Most clients experience these or other life-changing "aha!" moments as side effects. However, this is not the reason or the focus of the GEMT session. The ultimate goal of GEMT is to facilitate the client's understanding that she is not a victim and is responsible for manifesting her ailment.

What is Disease?

Disease is a dis-ease caused by negative perceptions. GEMT views ailments as symptoms or effects, not the cause of the disease. All pain and disease originate in the mind, specifically in the beliefs/perceptions of the subconscious, and the body is used to store negative emotions. The body, obedient to the messages from the subconscious mind, in turn creates pain, ailments, or pain-free perfect health.

People seek help with old issues, even if the symptoms are new. Overreaction to a situation indicates a re-stimulation of a core victimhood issue. Constant negative thinking with strong negative emotions about a situation or a past event sends a message to the subconscious to create the pain and ailment, so the emotion is physically manifested for the conscious mind's awareness. Dis-ease creates dis-comfort, and negative beliefs show up as symptoms.

In GEMT, manifested disease is cherished for its emotional aspects which are the key indicators to finding the core misperception. Beyond that, defining, analyzing or focusing on the facets or discord of a disease is unnecessary, and may have the adverse effect of giving it deeper roots. The only misperception GEMT focuses is that of victimhood. Once the client owns the disease, it is transmuted, healing the client of what we call "Victim Disease," the dis-ease associated with perceiving yourself as a victim. Regardless of the ailment and for the purpose of a GEMT session, we simply say, "**disease is an effect of misperception.**"

What is Healing?

There are many definitions of healing, all of which share a common theme. Common dictionary definitions include

- to make free from injury or disease
- to make sound or whole
- the process of making or becoming well or healthy again
- to cause (an undesirable condition) to be overcome
- to patch up or correct (a breach or division)
- to reconcile, or bring to an end or conclusion to, conflicts between people or groups
- to restore to original purity or integrity

Going beyond dictionary definitions, healing is the bringing of ease to where there is dis-ease, and healing cannot occur without recognizing the presence of the dis-ease. We can think of healing as a pendulum swinging from dis-ease to wellness or wholeness.

We get a deeper definition of healing from the article "*The Meaning of Healing: Transcending Suffering*," by Thomas R. Egnew, EdD, LICSW. for which seven allopathic physicians were interviewed.

In this article, healing was defined in the following terms:

- "Developing a sense of personal wholeness that involves physical, mental, emotional, social and spiritual aspects of human experience."
- "You can be healed and still have a physically sick body."
- "It's possible to be in health and to be healed without being cured."

The study concludes with this definition: "Healing is the personal experience of the transcendence of suffering." The healing occurs once the life story is improved and/or the meaning of the suffering is found and is independent from the physical ailment. The study also defines a healer by stating, "Healing is related to wholeness, and wholeness is experienced in connection with others.... A healer is somebody who's going to help you make those connections." This deeper definition of healing expands on the dictionary theme of moving away from suffering and toward wholeness by adding that healing is beyond the body and the meaning of the suffering needs to be found.

The definition of wholeness is derived from the word holistic and shares the root word for 'holy,' as in "spiritually pure or whole." Holistic health is about caring for the health of the whole person, including spiritual health. We get an even deeper definition of healing from the spiritual text of "A Course In Miracles":

- "Healing involves an understanding of what the illusion of sickness is for. Healing is impossible without this."

- "Healing is accomplished the instant the sufferer no longer sees any value in pain."
- "What is the single requisite for this shift in perception? It is simply this; the recognition that sickness is of the mind and has nothing to do with the body."
- "Healing and Atonement are not related; they are identical."

The spiritual definition of healing continues to expand on the dictionary and physician definitions, and includes the idea that suffering comes from the perception of being separate from who or what is victimizing. Healing is a decision of the mind to shift perception, and healing and atonement are one and the same. The decision-maker is the creator and Atonement (At-One-Ment) is One with The Creator and All That Is.

In consideration of the dictionary, physician, and spiritual definitions, we can define healing as stepping away from suffering while stepping toward wholeness through this shift in perception. If we consider that a creator must assume responsibility for what it creates, and that victim and sufferer are one and the same, GEMT introduces the concept that a shift in perception from victimhood to self-responsibility produces the quintessential onset for self-healing. Because we all have free will, every person has the right to choose to be healed or not, which makes all healing self-healing. Unlike some modalities, you need not be a licensed acupuncturist or mental health professional to be a GEMT practitioner. We define *healer* as someone who facilitates healing, which is essentially, all of us. ***Healing is a shift in perception away from suffering and toward wholeness.***

The Problem GEMT Solves

One issue with other modalities is that something other than the client's mind, such as a practitioner or a pill, can heal her. Even if the client chooses to believe this, it is inaccurate, misleading and disempowering. GEMT solves this problem by helping the client see that she is healing herself and is an active participant in the healing process. GEMT views past events as perfect and brilliant creations of the client and is one of the ways it differs from other modalities.

Clients might prefer a GEMT session because the practitioner:
- Exerts minimal personality, keeping the focus on the client
- Encourages mindful participation
- Sees ailments and symptoms as good and valuable
- Empathetically sees misperceptions as normal
- Accepts the client as right where she should be
- Sees everything as right, normal, and even brilliant
- Recognizes the client as powerful beyond comprehension
- Reminds the client that she is the creator of her own experience
- Reminds the client that nothing would exist unless it had value
- Finds great value in the client's unresolved issues
- Sees herself as a facilitator for the client to heal herself
- Does not interfere with the client's free will to choose sickness *or* health.

Clients inherently know they don't want a practitioner adding to their disease by having a negative perspective, seeing them as a victim or weak, disagreeing with their manifestations, seeing something wrong about them, having a problem that needs to be fixed, or believing that they are unable to heal themselves. We do not carelessly remove any ailment or discomfort with disregard to why it was manifested in the first place, or put our issues on a client, or take credit for healing. GEMT is in alignment with the spiritual idea of oneness and creates a healing shift in both the client and practitioner.

GEMT Compared to Hypnotherapy

Similar to hypnotherapy, when practicing GEMT we use our imagination to promote healing while the client is in a tranquil state. Though there are similarities to Conversational Hypnosis, GEMT is considered a cognitive therapy. Instead of a hypnotic deep trance, during GEMT the client bilaterally taps on meridian points to create a light alpha state or relaxed conscious state. Also, instead of being passive to the practitioner's dialog as in hypnosis, the client and practitioner repeat each other while the practitioner attempts to understand what it's like to have the dis-ease from the client's perspective. It has been said that "what Milton Erickson is to hypnosis, GEMT is to tapping modalities."

GEMT Compared to EFT

EFT is an excellent exposure-based therapy that resolves anxiety issues (fears, phobias, PTSD and the like) with a simple formula of generic statements most anyone can follow. Although GEMT and EFT share the same tapping points, GEMT uses both hands alternating on the same meridian point on both sides of the body in a left-right-left-right fashion. This activates bilateral stimulation, which is a process that stimulates both sides of the brain, increasing interhemispheric communication, and is used to help the client recall and process memories that produce fear or other toxic emotions.

In GEMT there are no generic self-acceptance statements such as the "Even though I have this (pain or ailment) ..." like there are in EFT. Such a statement would imply a devaluing of the pain or ailment. GEMT differs from EFT in that the client and practitioner will thank the ailment and the people involved for bringing the opportunity for healing a difficult event from the past. Some EFT related methods fabricate comforting memories to neutralize painful ones which gives relief yet maintains the victimhood perception. GEMT leaves traumatic memories intact seeing them as perfectly chosen catalyst events for specific evolutionary growth and healing. In EFT the client repeats what the practitioner says, yet in GEMT the practitioner also repeats what the client says and encourages the client to lead the conversation. The EFT discovery statement is "The cause of all negative emotions is a disruption in the body's energy system." implying the body is responsible for negative emotions. GEMT uses the hypnotherapy version: "Negative emotions are stored as disruptions in the body's energy system."

The GEMT approach to healing is philosophy based on the idea that the traumatic event is not a mistake, it was chosen. Using imagination and subtle logic, GEMT helps clients transform their perception of victimhood to the perception of power, responsibility, and purpose. GEMT makes no direct changes to the discomfort of dis-ease and only helps the client uncover the value of the dis-ease, seeing it as a teacher for mastering self-responsibility. GEMT does not solve traumatic problems and only recognizes one issue which is the illusion of separation or what we call Victim Disease. This makes GEMT a unique modality.

Bob's client Ms. M

Ms. M. was in desperate need of dental work, but due to a paralyzing fear, she avoided the dentist for almost 20 years. Just mentioning the dentist would cause cold sores in her mouth. Rather than face her fear, she endured agonizing tooth pain. Eventually, she sought help. She tried other tapping modalities, but they didn't work for her. By the time she came to me she was distraught and desperate to find the root cause of her fear.

Prior to our GEMT session Ms. M's fear level was a 10 on a 0 to 10 scale, and she was often brought to tears due to the pain in her mouth and her fear of the dentist. During the session, we focused on the value of the fear and that it served a purpose in her life. This shift in perspective allowed her to relax and regress to being 6 years old, crying in excruciating pain while a dentist drilled the wrong tooth without anesthesia. We discovered that the source of the pain was from the emotional trauma of feeling like a victim. No one believed she was in pain until the dentist discovered later it was the wrong tooth. The incident was framed around the idea that this experience was helpful to her for an unknown reason. Eventually, she realized that this traumatic experience taught her to be more truthful and vocal when she needs help. We thanked her childhood dentist for playing the perfect role and helping her learn this lesson. She called three days later and reported that she was able to see a dentist and have the necessary work done. She felt empowered and relaxed in the dentist chair and the discomfort was tolerable. The dentist even commented about what a great patient she was.

Quiz – Part 1

1) Why is "Meridian Tapping" used as part of the modality name rather than "desensitization" or "emotional anesthesia"?
   a) It discloses that GEMT is similar to other tapping modalities.
   b) It is the meridian tapping that does the healing.
   c) The act of tapping creates a mirroring and matching opportunity which helps build rapport.
   d) Practitioners must be licensed acupuncturists or mental health professionals.

2) GEMT differs from other modalities because
   a) It focuses on healing the reaction to the disease, not the disease itself.
   b) Instead of forgiving, the ailment and people involved are thanked.
   c) Past events are viewed as perfect and brilliant creations of the client.
   d) All the above

3) How does GEMT view disease?
   a) An effect of misperception.
   b) Cherished for its emotional aspects.
   c) Defining, analyzing or focusing on its facets or discord is unnecessary.
   d) All the above.

PART 2 – The GEMT Approach to Healing

"No problem can be solved from the same level of consciousness [or subconsciousness – ed.] that created it." — Albert Einstein

Diagnosing, Curing, and Healing

The medical profession defines diagnosis as the identification of an illness based on its symptoms and defines curing as the declaration of health based on the absence of symptoms. Healing, on the other hand, is not the removal or cessation of symptoms but rather a restoration of wholeness comparatively better than before the onset of dis-ease. As a GEMT practitioner, you can neither diagnose nor claim to cure any illness. However, GEMT has been shown to influence healing far beyond the level of health that existed prior to the onset of a diagnosed disease.

Misbeliefs

The two most common misbeliefs created from childhood source issues are "not enough" ("not good enough," "not smart enough," etc.) and "unlovable" ("hated," "ignored," etc.). In the language of a session, these can be reduced to the terms 'criticized' and 'disliked,' respectively. Knowing which misbelief exists can speed up the process of finding value in the difficult situation by virtue of how the client grew from the experience.

For example, if the childhood source issue was "I am not enough," the value might be how they grew to be more accepting of self and others, with less of a need to prove worthiness. If feeling "unlovable" was the issue, the value might be that she has grown in her self-love, learned to rely less on others to feel love, and increased her unconditional love for others.

All Emotional Reactions Are Learned

The way we react makes us all unique. No two people react to the same event the same way. When we experience something for the first time, we might react with a fear of the unknown, yet even then we have created that fear from a prior event. The emotion of a current disease is often caused by an overreaction learned in childhood prior to the development of reasoning skills. When a particular event is difficult for a client, we want to return to the time when the client first learned to react to a similar event in a negative way (fear, sadness, anger, etc.) When we update the reaction to the original event, reactions for all subsequent similar events change. This is why we give little attention to the current situation and instead use it as a direct path to address childhood traumatic misperceptions and misbeliefs.

Victim Disease

What we call "Victim Disease" is the dis-ease that comes from a perception of victimhood and seems to be at the core of negative emotions and manifested disease. This disempowering perception is the cause of blame, resentment, judgement, condemnation and retaliation, and at the root of hatred and unrest. When we allow conditions outside ourselves to dictate how we think or feel, it can ultimately result in some form of dis-ease. The easiest, simplest and immediate resolution of Victim Disease is to take responsibility for all existing conditions. GEMT focuses on overturning the perception of victimhood, so the client can decide whether or not to keep an ailment. This is the reason the practitioner guides the client to the value of what exists and does not focus on changing, modifying or eliminating the ailment. Influencing the client's decision to remove, change or modify an ailment she has created indicates judgment and disempowers her by interfering with her free will. Though Victim Disease is rampant, it is quickly healed with an empathetic approach and an acceptance of what is as the creator.

The Vibration Scale of Emotions

We often use the term 'vibration' when explaining levels on an emotional scale, because it seems to be more fitting than using the terms emotional energy or mood. The phrase 'raise our vibration' essentially means we are attempting to experience a more vitalizing emotion. There are a few popular emotional vibration scales, such as the "scale of emotions" from the book *Ask and It Is Given*, by Esther Hicks, which has 22 levels, and "Map of Consciousness" from the book *Power vs. Force,* by David R. Hawkins, M.D., Ph.D., which has 17 levels. For GEMT, we have defined a simpler emotional vibration scale with 7 levels.

The GEMT Vibration Scale of Emotions

> 7 - Love/Appreciation/Joy/Empowerment (*Creator*)
> 6 - Happiness/Gratefulness/Passion
> 5 - Hopefulness/Optimism/Enthusiasm
> 4 - Contentment/Satisfaction/Boredom
> 3 - Blame/Worry/Doubt
> 2 - Anger/Hatred/Revenge
> 1 - Fear/Shame/Guilt/Hopelessness (*Victim*)

Prior to the start of a GEMT session, we attempt to raise the client's vibration as high as possible by asking her to imagine conditions that will generate the emotions of love, appreciation, joy and empowerment. The higher the emotional vibration, the greater chance she has of becoming aware that she is the creator of her own life experiences. Though raising the client's vibration will often cause her to choose a different issue to work on, it can be seen as emotionally relevant to the original issue.

It is important to note that blame, anger, revenge, and hatred are higher emotional vibrations than guilt. It feels better to blame someone else, or even hate them, than to deal with feelings of guilt. However, healing guilt has the effect of cancelling the blame, anger, revenge and hatred used to mask the guilt.

Subjective Units of Distress Scale

The Subjective Units of Distress Scale (SUDS – also called Subjective Units of Disturbance Scale) uses 0 to 10 as a benchmark for measuring the subjective intensity of distress the client is feeling in that moment. The individual conducts a self-assessment and communicates the SUDS number to the practitioner, establishing the initial degree of discomfort. Reassessment at the end of the session is important for the realization that healing has occurred.

10 - Feeling unbearably bad, beside yourself, out of control as in a nervous breakdown, overwhelmed, at the end of your rope. Feeling so upset that you don't want to talk because no one could possibly understand your agitation.

9 - Feeling desperate. What most people call a 10 is actually a 9. Feeling extremely freaked out to the point that it almost feels unbearable. Feeling afraid of losing control of your emotions.

8 - Freaking out. The beginning of alienation.

7 - Starting to freak out, on the edge of some definitely bad feelings. You can maintain control with difficulty.

6 - Feeling bad to the point that you begin to think something ought to be done about the way you feel.

5 - Moderately upset, uncomfortable. Unpleasant feelings are still manageable with some effort.

4 - Somewhat upset to the point that you cannot easily ignore an unpleasant thought.

3 - Mildly upset. Worried, bothered to the point that you notice it.

2 - A little bit upset, but not noticeable unless you took care to pay attention to your feelings and then realize, "yes there is something bothering me."

1 - No acute distress and feeling basically good. If you took special effort you might feel something unpleasant but not much.

0 - Peace, serenity, total relief. No anxiety of any kind about any particular issue.

Quantifying Success

Quantifying success plays an important role in both healing and the client-practitioner relationship. We use SUDS (Subjective Units of Distress or Disturbance Scale, 0–10) to encourage the client to subjectively indicate the level of success of a session, though frequently most of the healing is felt in the days after the session. Before beginning a session, establish a SUDS level of intensity with the client. Then, measure SUDS again at the end of the session. This enables both the practitioner and the client to evaluate their progress.

Some benefits for measuring SUDS before and after a session:

- Affirms to the client's subconscious mind that healing has occurred
- Gives motivation to the subconscious to continue healing beyond the session
- Adds to the client's belief that this type of healing works
- Opens the client's mind to how she can heal herself
- Provides an indication as to where the client is with the issue
- Helps convince that the session was worthwhile
- SUDS numbers might be the only point of success the client remembers
- Increases the client's faith in the healing process
- Adds to the practitioner's influence in further sessions

Quantifying success is important in helping the subconscious recognize and accept a deep level of healing.

Desensitization Therapies and Meridian Tapping

Desensitization therapies are widely known as some of the most effective therapy techniques to help people overcome anxiety and phobias. These exposure-based techniques either relax or distract the client while they are being exposed to the feared object or situation. Our experiences disallow us from concurring with the claims that desensitization therapies alone can permanently remove negative emotions, cure diseases, and even forgive by tapping on forgiveness meridian points (pinky and index fingers). Aside from that, desensitization is essentially "emotional anesthesia," and has been one of the great breakthroughs in cognitive therapeutic healing, bringing life-changing results by allowing the client to calmly reevaluate intense past experiences.

While all desensitization therapies expose the client to the fear object and/or situation either by thinking about it or through actual exposure, the techniques differ in calming methods.

- **Systematic Desensitization** – Deep Breathing
- **Flooding** – Progressive Muscle Relaxation
- **Immersion Therapy** – Tighten/Release Muscle Relaxation
- **Bilateral Stimulation (BLS)** – Visual, Auditory or Tactile
- **Eye Movement Desensitization and Reprocessing (EMDR)** – Visual Bilateral
- **Thought Field Therapy (TFT)** – Energy Balance by Meridian Tapping
- **Emotional Freedom Technique (EFT)** – Energy Balance by Meridian Tapping

All desensitization therapies have proven to give temporary relief of fears, phobias and painful memories so they can be confronted with minimal discomfort. Because exposure-based techniques can be so straightforward, recipe formulas have been created so anyone can quickly resolve their fears and phobias by following specific steps. Yet resolving anger and forgiveness issues often becomes more complex and elusive when using recipes.

Just as desensitization by itself does not resolve or heal fear, it also does not heal anger or sadness issues because healing is a change in perception. Consider the analogy of using a potholder for a short time to take a hot pan out of an oven so it can cool. GEMT uses bilateral meridian tapping for emotional anesthesia (potholder) to view a normally painful situation (hot pan) so the perception about it can be changed (cooled down). Relief is not healing but can allow for a change in perception which does heal.

GEMT chooses to use Meridian Tapping for desensitization, not only because it balances the body's energy system; it also allows the practitioner and client to mirror each other. GEMT also incorporates tactile bilateral stimulation by alternating with one tap on the right side of the body, then one tap on the left side. Each specific acupressure point is self-tapped with fingertips at a rate of about 2 taps per second while focusing on reprocessing traumatic events.

Bilateral Meridian Tapping achieves the following:

- Desensitizes client to alleviate defensiveness
- Reduces anxiety
- Creates the effect of emotional anesthesia
- Decreases discomfort by balancing the body's energy system
- Affects the nervous system to induce the light trance alpha state
- Creates practitioner/client mirroring for increased client trust
- Allows the client to physically participate in the process of changing perceptions

There has been some confusion about whether tapping alone can resolve emotional issues. For clarity, the body cannot heal the mind; let us be mindful not to give our power away to the body's energy system. Meridian tapping itself does not do the healing. It is and will always be mind over matter in the mind-body connection, never the reverse.

Bilateral Meridian Tapping Points

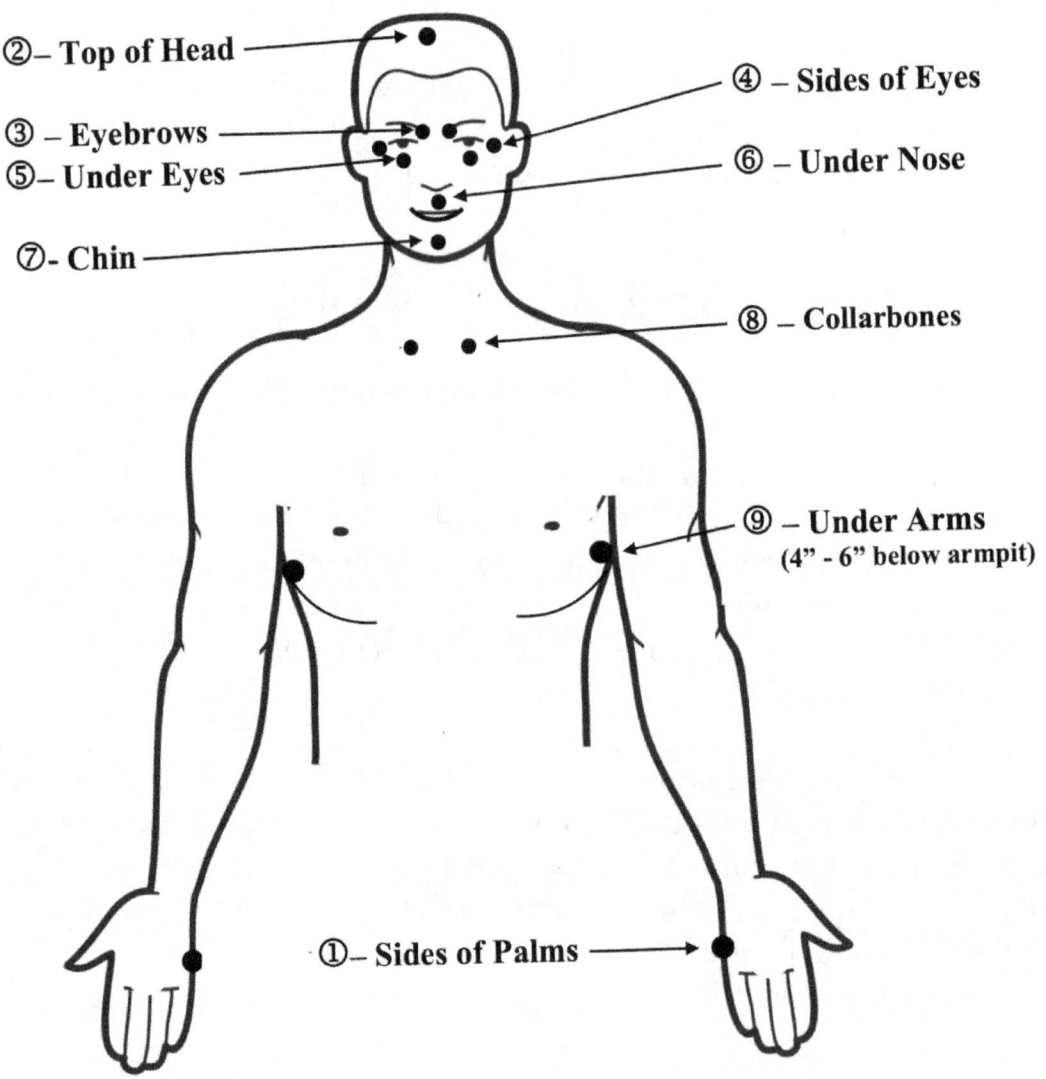

②– Top of Head

③ – Eyebrows

⑤– Under Eyes

⑦- Chin

④ – Sides of Eyes

⑥ – Under Nose

⑧ – Collarbones

⑨ – Under Arms
(4" - 6" below armpit)

①– Sides of Palms

1. **Side of Palm Point** (Small Intestine Meridian) – Located on the soft fleshy part of the hand, between the base of the little finger and the wrist. The right side of the palm is used to tap the left side of the palm so that both Sides of Palm points are stimulated by tapping on each other.
2. **Top of Head Point** ("Hundred Meeting Points" Meridian) – Located at the top of the head. An important energy center where many meridians meet at the top of the head, it is also in the area of the Crown Chakra, which is a spiritual energy center. This area awakens the entire energy system and encourages the body-mind to pay attention to what we are about to address. This point is highly sensitive, and it is important to be very gentle when tapping.
3. **Eyebrow Point** (Bladder Meridian) – Located at the beginning of the eyebrow, just up and over from the bridge of the nose.
4. **Side of Eye Point** (Gall Bladder Meridian) – Located on the bony protrusion at the leading edge of the temple and the end of the eyebrow.
5. **Under Eye Point** (Stomach Meridian) – Located on the bone underneath the eye about an inch directly under the pupil.
6. **Under Nose Point** (Governing Meridian) – Located under the nose, in the little crevice above the upper lip.
7. **Chin Point** (Central Meridian) – Located just under the bottom lip, in the depression between the lip and the chin.
8. **Collarbone Point** (Kidney Meridian – Adrenal Gland Function) – Located just below the knob of the collarbone and next to the depression below the Adam's apple.
9. **Under Arm Point** (Spleen Meridian) – Located about four to six inches directly below the armpit.

Using both hands, meridian points on both sides of the body are alternatingly tapped, one tap on the right side on the body then one tap on the left. This incorporates tactile bilateral stimulation by the action of hand movement as well as the stimulation of the meridian point. Under the nose, chin and top of the head, both hands are used on the same point in an alternating fashion. By a slight back-and-forth and clockwise-counterclockwise rotation, the left and right sides of the palms can also create a subtle bilateral stimulation. Each meridian point is tapped seven to ten times at a rate of about two taps per second each. If a client has only one usable hand, that hand taps seven to ten times on the point on one side of the body, then taps the point on the other side of the body to incorporate bilateral stimulation with the least amount of distraction.

How to Achieve Maximum Emotional Anesthesia

Defensiveness is a common reaction when a client's perceptions and beliefs are logically challenged to be misperceptions and misbeliefs. The less defensive the client, the more open she is to accept new perceptions. The greater the emotional anesthesia produced by meridian tapping, the greater the reduction in defensiveness for a "shift" happening. Ideally, all nine meridian points would be continually stimulated throughout the session to achieve the maximum emotional anesthesia. However, stimulation is managed by monitoring the time spent tapping at each meridian while the other eight points go untapped. It can take as little as four taps to stimulate a meridian point and achieve noticeable effects, and the sooner the tapping is returned to each meridian point, the better. GEMT already incorporates tactile bilateral stimulation by alternating a tap on the right side of the body then a tap on the left, such that the meridian point on each side of the body ideally gets seven to ten taps at about two taps per second before moving to the next. It is important to keep in mind that the level of emotional anesthesia correlates to how many points are kept stimulated.

Adding the following techniques from other desensitization therapies while tapping can help increase emotional anesthesia when the client's defensiveness is high.

- **Side-to-Side Eye Movement** – from Visual Bilateral Stimulation
- **Deep Breathing** – from Systematic Desensitization
- **Tighten/Release Muscle Relaxation** – from Immersion Therapy

Mirroring Matching Rapport

Milton Erickson, M.D. is largely credited as the first to use the rapport building techniques of mirroring and matching as a part of his conversational hypnosis. His hypnotic techniques allowed him to successfully offer suggestions and perspectives to his clients without formally inducing trance. In GEMT, as the client focuses on tapping the same meridian points as the practitioner, she is also inadvertently mirroring the practitioner. When the client and practitioner repeat each other's words, they are now also matching each other. Once mirroring and matching rapport has been established, the practitioner can guide the client to an empowering perspective.

The Healing Power of Empathy

We live in a world of free will, contrast, chaos and uncertainty, which often creates difficult situations and can result in people experiencing negative and toxic emotions. Much of the suffering comes from a feeling of being a victim of separation or being singled out. Being assured that she is not alone, unusual, weird, or an outcast brings normalcy and comfort to the client and ease to the session. Empathy heals in its own right. This is demonstrated by the significant impact on arachnophobia with the simple statement to a phobic client, "We are all afraid of spiders at some level." An empathetic statement does not have to be true to have the effects of healing. Empathy is the opposite of judgement.

Your purpose is to find value in a client's decision made during a stressful time, not to criticize the client's ability to make decisions nor to make any on behalf of the client. The practitioner knows that the client has the ability to make better decisions now, while in a safe empathetic conversation, than during that stressful time earlier in life, which is the source of the current issue for which she needs help. The statement "You don't need to be afraid of the thing you were afraid of when you were five" may seem helpful, yet the deep healing of the childhood reaction would come from a statement more like, "Anyone would be afraid of that at five, and it's quite understandable how some of that fear would still exist today." The latter empathetic statement, accompanied by the emotional anesthesia of tapping, provides the ease and safety for the subconscious mind to accept a new perception.

As healers, we place a high importance on emotions because of their powerful effect on health and wellness. Often, when someone overreacts and turns to us for comfort, we unconsciously dismiss her reaction and share our elevated perspective about the situation, which can add to her dis-ease. This is the time to empathize and not the best time to advise, mediate, problem-solve, or remind her there are many ways to perceive a situation. If we fall into the trap of trying to "teach" her to see it our way or set aside her feelings and empathize with those she believes have hurt her, we invalidate her and her feelings. This approach harms by adding to her dis-ease, and unaddressed feelings are stored as negative emotions in the body's energy system, most likely to resurface later.

In the 1895 poem by Mary T. Lathrap, originally titled "*Judge Softly*," later titled "*Walk a Mile in His Moccasins*," we are reminded to practice empathy by first walking a mile in someone's shoes before judging them.

> *"Just for a moment, slip into his mind and traditions*
> *And see the world through his spirit and eyes*
> *Before you cast a stone or falsely judge his conditions."*

It is the same for a GEMT session; we essentially set out to empathetically walk a mile in the client's shoes.

An Empathetic Approach Has Three Major Benefits
1. The practitioner gains greater influence to guide the client.
2. The practitioner gains a better understanding of the client's issue.
3. The client gains a new perspective by "seeing" her issue in the practitioner.

Empathy vs. Sympathy

In general, empathy is when we understand, share, and are sensitive to the feelings of another. Sympathy is when we feel compassion or sorrow for the hardships experienced by another. In GEMT, both sympathy and empathy agree with the emotion. However, empathy may or may not be in agreement with the perspective that created it. Empathy can heal with its understanding, but sympathy could be considered harmful when it perceives or judges a situation as bad. A literal empathetic statement might be "I agree with your emotions because I understand your perspective." A literal sympathetic statement would be "I agree with your emotions because I share the same perspective."

The Use of Empathy in a GEMT Session

An empathetic perspective allows the practitioner to validate the client's emotion by somewhat experiencing it in the session while keeping the emotional focus on the client.

Components of Empathy

- Client feels heard by the practitioner.
- Practitioner is in agreement with what has been manifested.
- Practitioner affirms the client's truth is correct from the client's point of view.
- Practitioner affirms the client's feelings are understandable and normal.
- Practitioner affirms the client's behavioral responses have been normal.
- Practitioner is at ease with where the client is now.

What manifests NOW is a product of the unchangeable past. What is changeable is the way we perceive it. As healers, we can influence healing by empathetically offering a new perspective to the client.

Emotional Agreement

It is a basic rule of life that we care for our own emotions first or we will not be emotionally available to others. Healing comes from empathizing, not advising, mediating or problem-solving. For example, it's best to first empathize with someone and validate her feelings, which allows her to calm herself before suggesting she be empathetic to another person.

Just listening can heal. Actively listening is letting her know she was heard and understood. Empathetic or empathic listening is active listening with validation, i.e., "It's ok to feel that way." GEMT takes it further by an emotional understanding that comes from agreeing with her emotions. To be in emotional agreement would be the highest level of empathy, i.e., "I would feel that way too if I were in your shoes." The highest level of empathetic healing is to fully validate the client by completely agreeing with her response and feelings about the situation. This is not difficult because emotions are never wrong from the perception of what created them and agreeing with them does not mean agreeing with the misperceptions. In an empathetic GEMT session, we listen, understand and are in agreement with her emotions.

A Review of Empathetic Responses

The following 3 scenarios are intended to illustrate the contrast between emotional agreement vs unintentional invalidation.

Father Forgets Fishing Trip
Your friend John, in his thirties, has been working on rebuilding a relationship with his father who abandoned the family when John was seven. Since reconnecting a few years ago, John's father has shown up for every event that John planned for them, except one. This time it was John's father's idea to spend the afternoon fishing in a nearby pond, and he had planned to pick up John at 1 pm.

At 2:30 John calls you, distraught; his father just texted that he forgot about the plans. John begins ranting that his father is inconsiderate, a lost cause, and does not care about him.

Unempathetic responses that invalidate John and his feelings:
   a) "Well, of course your father cares about you."
   b) "Overall, the relationship with your father has been improving, right?"
   c) "Maybe your father has a lot going on right now."

Empathetic and healing responses that validate John and his feelings:
   a) "You are right to be upset! That is just plain wrong and inconsiderate."
   b) "That would make anyone get upset and feel hurt."
   c) "I would feel the same way if I experienced what you went through."

Passed Up for Lead Role
Nancy, the 10-year-old daughter of a neighborhood friend, frequently visits your home to make cookies and sew. Recently Nancy has been talking about her quest to get the lead role in the upcoming school play and feels that she is the director's first choice for the lead role. However, you are friends with the director, Beth, and have heard her perspective on the children auditioning for the parts.

When Nancy finds out she was chosen for a smaller role in the play, she is disappointed and upset. She thinks Beth misled her into believing she would get the lead role just to trick her into the smaller role.

Unempathetic responses that invalidate Nancy and her feelings:
   a) "I know Beth is a good director, so there must be a reason for her decision."
   b) "Maybe Beth needed someone strong to play that smaller role."
   c) "Maybe Beth did not see enough of your audition."

Empathetic and healing responses that validate Nancy and her feelings:
   a) "You are absolutely right to feel this way."
   b) "Anyone would be upset at that. No one likes feeling misled."
   c) "I would be disappointed too."

Movers are a No-Show

Your friend Bill owns a moving company and is regularly looking for work. Mary, an acquaintance at your office, is asking around for referrals for moving companies. The next day in the office break room you recommend Bill's moving company to Mary. Bill calls you later that evening to thank you for the referral.

A month later, Mary comes by your office very upset, explaining that Bill's moving company did not show up for the move. In her state of anger, she rants about Bill's unprofessionalism and points out that you were the one who recommended him.

Unempathetic responses that invalidate Mary and her feelings:
   a) "I wonder why that happened. What was Bill's excuse for this?"
   b) "I know Bill has been taking on a lot of extra work recently."
   c) "This is unexpected. Bill has a great track record."

Empathetic and healing responses that validate Mary and her feelings:
   a) "Wow! That is shocking and extremely upsetting!"
   b) "You are absolutely right! That is extremely unprofessional."
   c) "I apologize for recommending Bill and I would be upset at me too."

The above scenarios demonstrate how to validate emotions, and how emotions are invalidated with common automatic responses. Invalidating or arguing with someone's emotions creates a problem; she feels unheard and thinks her feelings are wrong when, in fact, they are not wrong. Through GEMT we see that emotions are a guidance system and correct for that person, in that moment, and though a person's perception may be inaccurate, the emotion that correlates to misperception is never wrong.

("Once you understand your own Emotional Guidance System, you will never again be confused about where you are in relationship to where you want to be. … Only when you pay attention to the way you feel can you guide yourself steadily toward your own goals." – Abraham Hicks)

Dismissing and devaluing emotions can cause dis-ease which can develop into a number of issues including illness, depression, violence and addiction. Simply validate the emotion first; it is easy to do and allows the person to feel at ease about those emotions. Nothing can change until we validate our feelings and accept where we are. Once validated there is no longer a need to protect those feelings, and healing can happen through a change in perception.

Empathetic Influence

As healers, all we can do is influence the healing of others, because all have free will and make their own choices. We are occasionally influenced by experts, successful people, and people we like and admire, but we are most influenced by the people who understand us. The strongest position of influence is one of empathy, because most people are only open to outside influence in correlation to their feelings of being understood. To have influence on another, empathy must be present, and the greater the empathy, the more powerful the influence. We choose a specialist to help because we believe they have the greatest empathy for our situation, not necessarily because of their qualifications. Life's most challenging experiences become the empathetic tools you can utilize as a GEMT practitioner.

GEMT focuses on the powerful empathetic approach to influence healing because healing begins as soon as the client feels at ease and understood.

Empathetic Bond

What we call empathetic bond is a unique type of rapport that is created when the client and practitioner are mirroring tapping points and repeating "I" statements. This is the cornerstone for influencing healing through

GEMT. In some cases, when the client and practitioner mirror their words and tapping points so closely, an observer might be unable to identify who is the client and who is the practitioner. This allows the client to somewhat see her ailment in someone else, feel at ease that she is not alone, and gives the practitioner empathetic influence to suggest valuable scenarios.

Dorthy's client Mr. A

Mr. A, referred to me by his doctor, was in so much physical pain throughout his body that he could barely move. None of the medical strategies were helpful in finding the source of his pain. They found nothing biological or physiological so his doctor, who determined the pain was psychosomatic, encouraged hypnotherapy. After just three or four hypnotherapy sessions, Mr. A experienced positive results until a business problem occurred. Then, the pain returned, tormenting him again.

I explained the process of GEMT, and he quickly agreed to try it after reporting his pain level at a 10 on a SUDS scale. Following the suggested steps for a session, we spoke of many things including his feelings about lying to his past business partner about why he wanted to end the partnership and who ultimately died of a heart attack. He discovered, during GEMT conversation, the emotion associated with his pain was guilt about lying to his partner.

Through the discovery process of GEMT he shared about an event long ago in Italy when he was five years old, and his father beat him mercilessly for lying. His subconscious mind had correlated guilt with physical pain, and the emotion of guilt produced pain throughout his body. Introducing the empathetic statement "All humans lie, either knowingly or unknowingly" produced an obvious relief and ease in his body. When we brought up the idea of "why would I choose a parent who would beat me so hard for lying?" he immediately stated, "Because I needed to be forced to stop the habit of lying, else people I love will get hurt." We thanked his father, his business partner, and the pain for helping him learn the most important lesson of his life.

Through the empathetic process of GEMT, his release of an old unconscious perception of being a victim, and his ultimate gratitude and forgiveness, his pain disappeared along with the original subconscious correlation.

Following GEMT with hypnosis, we anchored the new knowledge and instilled post-hypnotic suggestions for management of responses. He is now and has been free from that pain for several years.

Do No Harm

The number one rule in healing is to "do no harm." Judging is the act of devaluing; however, everything that exists has value. Judgment is harmful when felt by a client seeking help. She needs your empathy, understanding and expertise, rather than added judgment. If you dislike, disagree or disapprove of the client's situation, you have formed a judgmental opinion and are trying to discard the valuable tool that the client has manifested and no longer acting in the best interest of the client. This also harms you as a practitioner because you are in dis-ease about someone else's use of free will over which you have no control. If your feelings are neutral about the client's situation, you are actually in resistance to it being "good" or a beneficial presence, an indication that there must be something about their unchangeable past with which you don't agree. In this case, you are in judgement and would be adding dis-ease to the client. When you see a problem in your client, then it becomes your problem, and you are not in acceptance of what is. Your goal is to accept things as they are. When you realize you feel emotionally neutral about a client's situation or disease, take the stance that there must be a major upside, but it is currently beyond comprehension. If you are unable to accomplish this, the session should end so the client is not harmed.

Instead of giving attention to what you think about the client, give attention to the client in the present moment and the rule to "do no harm."

A Review of Being Non-Judgmental

As an example, we might have expectations for our friends to be supportive when others might not be. Let's say you started a hobby painting landscapes and decided to take a beginning painting course. Your first painting might not be so great in classic terms, yet you are proud of your creation because it symbolizes trying a hobby you were interested in. You show it to your friend with the expectation that she will be encouraging and will find some value or good quality about your painting, not criticize it. Why else would you show it to your friend? You might even feel that your friend's encouraging remarks might help counterbalance your own feelings of criticism and dis-ease about your creation.

However, your friend's, or anyone's criticism could add to your dis-ease about your creation. You might even consider hiding your novice paintings to avoid unsolicited criticisms from those who might not be so supportive and evade the added stress and effort of defending your creation with "This is where I am right now: better than yesterday, not as good as tomorrow."

Like our paintings, we are the creators of our life situations. Most of us are far from mastering life, so our situations might not look good overall and can be difficult to hide. To be a non-judgmental friend is to find some value or good quality about a friend's situation to bring ease and healing. This is extremely important because the dis-ease about life situations is what creates illness. As healers, we bring ease to a client's life situations as if they were a novice painter, by letting go of the role of Judge and returning to our number one rule: Do No Harm.

No Problem-Solving Required

Most clients are seeking help dealing with their current issues even though they have the reasoning abilities to resolve them on their own. Helping clients understand their current issues through reasoning, even with the most enlightening philosophy, won't fully resolve their issue or explain their reaction to it. This is because the source of the problem is stimulated by a traumatic memory when the client did not have the coping skills to handle the event. This is why there is nothing wrong with the client's situation and why we don't waste time trying to fix it. We view the client's current situation as an exciting opportunity to quickly address unresolved childhood trauma, which has the benefit of resolving their current issue.

Want What is Best for Your Client

As a GEMT practitioner, you cannot know what is best for your client, because of the limited knowledge and personal perspective you have of the client's situation. Having preconceived ideas about the client prior to the session increases the risk of drawing erroneous conclusions, producing misdirected advice, and bringing focus to what the practitioner wants to have happen, rather than what the situation calls for, or what the client needs. You do not need to decide what is best for the client, except of course, to want the best for your client. When you trust the process, empty of expectations, you are also presenting or bringing about the "so what" attitude concerning an old issue, which is also an integral part of the healing process. To help you keep mindful of this, say to your client quietly in your mind "I want what is best for you, but I have no idea what that is."

Some "wanted outcome" from the practitioner is a distraction from truly being present with the client. "Wants" of the practitioner create expectations for the client, and these expectations can be a precursor to judgment. When that happens, the client feels it. "Wants" are usually specific, and any "want" from the practitioner will only limit the options for the client, because that specific "want" tends to rule out all other possibilities and directions. It is our opinion that in order to be of the most appropriate service, the practitioner must simply desire to serve the client without any conditions put on that desire. A practitioner only wants what is best for her client and also knows she does not know what that is. Only tapping and an empathetic conversation will lead the client and practitioner to what is best for the client. Even the client doesn't know what will be revealed and resolved. That's the adventure.

Understanding and Approaching the Client

The practitioner, at ease with "what is," views the client as normal and fine, regardless of her issue. The client, in a state of dis-ease possibly because she feels separate from the world around her, and/or is suffering from the misbelief she is not enough, has created subconscious misperceptions of herself as a victim. These are key points to reverse at every opportunity. Because most people dislike viewing themselves as a victim, the conscious awareness of this perception can help in the acceptance of responsibility for it. Also, by virtue of the client seeking help, great healing potential is already established. Your genuine curiosity as to why your client is not reacting to her issue with a "so what" attitude will reveal it as a stimulation of a past unresolved childhood event when she first began to perceive herself as a victim.

In a GEMT session the practitioner becomes a tool of the client for self-discovery. It's best to allow your client's personality to dominate the session and the sooner the session begins, the easier it is to stay focused on her. To help stay focused, say your client's name at the beginning of the session, as in, "I'm so happy to work with you today, Nancy." This is fundamental to establishing the Empathetic Bond, which is the most powerful factor for influencing healing. It is also important to repeat what your client says, verbatim, because her choice of words is one of her most identifying characteristics.

How to Perceive the Client

GEMT is just one of the many healing modalities that can help achieve amazing results for the clients of both new and experienced practitioners. It is not uncommon for new practitioners to develop a sense of pride in their ability to successfully facilitate healing. However, if this pride goes unchecked it can negatively affect the way a client is perceived during a session. If the client is viewed as someone who needs your help to solve her problems or who has an ailment you are confident you can remove; the session is now less about what is best for the client and more about validating yourself as a successful healer. New practitioners who develop this unconscious perspective of viewing a client as another person who will validate how great a healer they are, often wonder why their client base is low. It is certainly best for both client and practitioner that the practitioner keeps her pride in check.

Even the kindest and most patient practitioners can bring dis-ease to clients, especially if they feel overly sympathetic when perceiving ailments as harmful to their clients. The only surefire way to allow the client to be at ease is for you to be at ease with her and her issue. Coddling a client with extra kindness can be harmful because it risks her thinking that you think she is helpless, weak or a victim, or that her manifestation is bad. Treat your clients as normal healthy individuals regardless of their issues, because each of us at our core is normal and healthy. You as the practitioner must be a non-judgmental observer, and view every client as unique, important and equal.

The most ideal way to perceive your client is that she is part of you and everything that exists. Think of that time, 13.8 billion years ago, when we were all in oneness as the Universe, and suddenly the Big Bang occurred. When that happened, the Universe separated and scattered itself like pieces of a jigsaw puzzle, with each piece unique, important and equal as a part of the original Oneness. From that perspective you can view your client, and anyone with whom she might have an issue, as one with the same single entity 13.8 billion years ago and an equally invaluable piece of the universal puzzle now. One way you might remind yourself of this is by using a phrase such as, "I am at Peace seeing her as an infinitely valuable Piece to the puzzle without which the Universe cannot be whole and complete."

Work on What the Client Is Ready to Resolve

Regardless of the primary reason the client is seeking help, in GEMT we focus first on what the client is ready to have happen. The easiest perspective for the client is the one seen from her highest vibration or mood. We first raise the vibration of the client, and then ask, "What would you like to work on today?" The response will be used later to start a conversation. Using this process provides clarity and empowers the client to choose from a higher vibration. Though clients sometimes change the focus of their session to something seemingly unrelated, both issues often share the same particular underlying emotion.

Recognize the Value of Disease and Discomfort

Why are there such things as pain and disease? Why does a person manifest any kind of ailment in the first place? The answer is the same for both: pain and ailments have value, and that value is letting us know we need to make corrections in our perceptions. The value of pain is that it is a calling for immediate attention of the conscious mind to take corrective action as soon as possible.

The value of a manifested disease brings awareness that the storage of negative emotions has now reached a critical level and the manifested disease holds all the information needed to heal an event from the past. When past events are resolved, the subconscious mind dissolves negative emotions, which allows the client to return to well-being. For this reason, we consistently thank the dis-ease for providing the opportunity for deep healing to occur.

Trauma and Reasoning

Experiencing trauma is a part of life. It is our reasoning ability, which does not develop until later in life, that brings it under control. As children without reasoning skills, we draw erroneous and inaccurate conclusions about ourselves based on our interpretation of traumatic events. We also begin to condemn others as a coping mechanism to protect ourselves. The easiest time to find and resolve these early childhood trauma misperceptions is when they resurface as difficult situations later in life.

GEMT guides the conversation back to "the" time when the client had an experience that caused a similar emotion to that of her current issue. If she remembers having a phobic overreaction to an event, then the reaction was learned from an experience that happened earlier. We have found that core issues and misperceptions originate prior to the development of reasoning skills, which typically begin developing around the age of 8.

Reversing Condemnation

We know that mistakes are a natural part of our learning process, but when we condemn someone, it impedes this learning. Condemning someone for making a mistake can create the perception of being "better" than that person or even having power over her. However, the one doing the condemning still maintains the associated negative emotions, and that can lead to dis-ease. Children who experience trauma often feel comfort in the power of condemning, especially when they feel like a victim and are not able to give someone the benefit of the doubt. They might also choose this power to counter the misperception of feeling "less than" or "not enough," such as "I had a bad father because his work was more important than family. He never came to my school events," as well as to compensate for something that did not happen, such as "I hate my parents because they wouldn't let me play after school." Children do not have the skills to find value in a difficult situation, nor are they able to perceive that they created the situation. Forgetting about the situation does not stop condemnation from resurfacing later in life as an ailment or strong negative emotional reactions.

This is why reevaluating early childhood issues that happened prior to the development of reasoning skills is one of the main components of GEMT. Once a person develops reasoning skills, she can reevaluate past situations and choose whether or not to continue to condemn. Forgiveness is the cessation of condemnation. On the occasion when a client argues, "If the difficult childhood trauma hadn't happened, then I wouldn't have to forgive," you can offer the idea that if she chooses to stop condemning, then she won't have to forgive. This reverses condemnation and is one of the key aspects of replacing the idea of victimhood with self-responsibility.

Why Acceptance is Needed to Heal

We often reject dis-ease by masking the symptoms and discomfort in an attempt to remedy a malfunctioning body. This may give us temporary relief only to re-manifest or morph into an even bigger health issue. This is because the subconscious mind that created the discomfort and dis-ease is working as it should, storing negative emotions in the body. The way to heal is to accept that there is a negative perception causing the dis-ease, not a body that needs correcting.

Relief is not healing, and remedies do not heal. Remedies often provide faster relief than healing though some form of the issue will most likely reappear when the effects of a remedy go away. Remedies can be harmful to the healing process because healing is impossible without discomfort. When there is an opportunity for healing, it is a great disservice to the client to take away the pain without offering a change in the perception that caused it in the first place. Once the client begins feeling relief, it is important for her to focus on accepting that she is the creator.

Why Self-Responsibility Is Needed for Complete Healing

There are people who do not make it a priority to heal themselves, just as there are people who do not make it a priority to clean their own home. When it's not a priority to keep a clean house, the responsibility for cleaning is often based on who created the mess, rather than who has to live with it. As in the resistance to cleaning someone else's mess, we tend to resist healing our dis-ease when we blame someone else for creating it. When we make someone else responsible for the cleaning/healing, it can never be fully cleaned or completely healed, and we will live in dis-ease with what we believe are the remnants of someone else's issue or mess. When we take full responsibility for the dis-ease and healing, healing is complete.

50

Clients suffering from pain or dis-ease want relief, yet some don't want to hear that they created the dis-ease. These clients struggle with the emotional element of victimhood masking their dis-ease. In some sessions the practitioner may ask the client, "What percentage of you does not want the dis-ease to go away?" If the client is not disturbed by the dis-ease, or is in agreement with it, or OK living with it, there is no victimhood to resolve, and healing can be done with decisions about perceived value. However, if victimhood is present, the client must first accept self-responsibility for the ailment before healing can be complete.

When we take full responsibility and ownership for our issues, cleanup becomes fast, easy and complete. What was previously considered someone else's mess now becomes our creation for the purpose of learning and growing through life's experiences. Whatever blemishes or stains remain become the trophies and diplomas of our accomplishment in self-empowerment, which is the core concept of GEMT. As the practitioner influences the overturning of the client's victimhood and suggests complete responsibility as Creator for the issue, the client feels the freedom to heal completely and quickly.

Tools that help the client take responsibility for the victimhood issue include emotional anesthesia from bilateral meridian tapping, accompanying empathetic "I" statements, building rapport from modeling and mirroring, and recognizing the value given to difficult situations. When the client understands that no issue can exist without her permission and without playing some role in it, however small, the tools of GEMT are no longer needed. The ultimate healing happens when the client accepts control over her life and makes adjustments as difficult situations arise, regardless of the perceived value.

Importance of Client Sobriety and Cognitive Coherence

With GEMT, it is imperative that the client is cognitively coherent and unimpaired while engaged in meridian tapping, as with most other therapies or cognitive procedures. When the human brain is affected by any toxic/impairing substance such as alcohol or drugs, that person cannot participate in the process of her healing. The time and energy spent in a session is wasted and is of very little or no value when the client is under the influence and unable to participate on all levels. When we participate in our own healing, mentally, physically and emotionally, the healing and shift occurs even more profoundly at the deepest levels within us. The client needs to experience the shift that happens, not be numb to it. When clients want to work on addiction issues, the GEMT practitioner is responsible for 2 things:

1. Prior to the session, inform of the 72-hour detoxification rule. (It takes at least 72 hours for the human body to detoxify after the last drink. Drugs can take many days or even weeks. DO NOT waste your time working with someone who is currently using!)
   a. Example: "I would love to work with you, and I have a rule that I only do a session with someone who has been clean and sober for at least 72 hours. Would you like to schedule your session for 4 days from today?"
2. Before beginning the session, ask if they are using today. (A good question to ask all clients and essential for an addict.)

Recognizing Stress as Dis-ease

What is Stress? Stress is our internal response to our perception of the world around us. As a victim our perceptions create our stress.

The definitions of stress are many:
- Mental, emotional, physical strain or tension
- A physical, chemical, or emotional factor that causes bodily or mental tension and is a factor in disease causation
- Stress typically is described as a negative concept that may impact one's mental and physical well-being

A few quotes about stress:
- "Stress is when you wake up screaming and realize you haven't fallen asleep yet." —Unknown
- "If your teeth are clenched and your fists are clenched, your lifespan is probably clenched." —Adabella Radici
- "We don't see things as they are, we see them as we are." -Anais Nin

Symptoms of Stress

Examples of behavioral symptoms of stress:
- Overeating
- Smoking
- Drinking (alcohol)
- Addictions (TV, electronic games, substances, etc.)
- Increased OCD (obsessive-compulsive disorder)
- Insomnia
- Depression
- _____
- _____

Examples of physical symptoms of stress:
- Pain
- Illness
- Anxiety attacks
- _____
- _____

Areas of Life That Contribute to Stress:
- Health Issues
- Relationships
- Job/Career
- Finances
- Self-perception
- _____
- _____

Stress and Your Body

- Stress is a part of life and not always problematic
- Stress is a major contributing factor to pain and dis-ease when it is constant and chronic
- Pain and dis-ease (and their symptoms) are signals from your body that you are not paying attention to something important, e.g.
  a. Indications of "burn-out"
  b. Subconscious sabotaging beliefs
  c. Immune system is compromised
  d. Unresolved negative emotions

Conditions and Issues that Can Be Indirectly Transformed with GEMT

As you become more proficient in the use of GEMT you will be adept enough to try it on many other conditions as well, e.g.

- Fears and Phobias
- Pain Management
- Weight Loss/Eating Disorders
- Children's Issues
- Addictions and Obsessions
- Allergy Relief/Allergies
- Trauma/Abuse
- Insomnia/Sleep Problems
- PTSD (Post Traumatic Stress Disorder)
- Asthma Relief
- Tension Headaches/Migraine Headaches
- Relationship Problems
- Vision Issues
- Learning and Study Problems
- Self-Esteem Issues
- Rage and Anger Management
- Performance Anxiety
- Depression

- Carpal Tunnel Syndrome
- ADD/ADHD (Attention Deficit Disorders)
- OCD (Obsessive Compulsive Disorder)
- High (or Low) Blood Pressure
- Diabetes/Neuropathy
- Fear of Flying
- Claustrophobia
- Agoraphobia
- Physical Manifestations

History of GEMT

Meridian tapping has roots in the ancient Chinese medicine of acupuncture, which uses needles to stimulate energy meridian pathways. Acupuncture has become more recognized and accepted by Western medicine for anesthesia and physical healing, and although it is a powerful physical healing technique, acupuncture was not developed to treat emotional problems.

The meridian tapping thread of "emotional acupressure" was first utilized by Dr. George Goodheart, who first learned about acupuncture in 1962. Shortly thereafter he studied acupuncture and introduced it into his own work called Applied Kinesiology, or "muscle testing." He found that he could obtain the same beneficial results simply by "tapping" on the meridians rather than using needles. In the 1970s, John Diamond, M.D., an Australian psychiatrist, added affirmations while tapping and called it "Behavioral Kinesiology." This began the "meridian-based therapies" and Energy Psychology, now known as GEMT. In the early 1980s, psychologist Dr. Roger Callahan learned Applied Kinesiology, studied the meridian system of acupuncture, and combined the use of "tapping" for emotional problems while focusing on the problem itself. Callahan discovered that his process would often permanently remove a fear or phobia. He outlined a series of specific tapping sequences he called "algorithms" or "Acutap" and created a technique called "Thought Field Therapy" or "TFT." achieving some remarkable results.

Brief Record of Energy Therapy

- 5000 BC – Neolithic people marked acupuncture treatment points
- 3000 BC – "Yellow Emperor" publishes text on acupuncture
- 1964 – Dr. George Goodheart: muscle-testing & Applied Kinesiology
- 1979 – John Diamond, MD: Behavioral Kinesiology. Used affirmations with tapping. Book: *Your Body Doesn't Lie*
- 1979 – Dr. Roger Callahan developed Thought Field Therapy (TFT). Used affirmations and tapping with a water-phobic client. Book: *Tapping the Healer Within*
- 1995 – Gary Craig developed Emotional Freedom Techniques (EFT)
- 1998 – Association for Meridian Energy Therapies (AMT) founded
- 1999 – Association for Comprehensive Energy Psychology (ACEP) founded
- 2010 – Gray Craig relinquished EFT to public domain
- 2011 – Robert Ranche and Dorthy Tyo create GEMT – Guided Empathy Meridian Tapping

The Discovery: 1980

Mary, a client of Dr. Callahan, saw him for over a year for severe water phobia and nightmares. One day she said she felt a nervousness in her stomach about the issue. Dr. Callahan tried tapping on the stomach meridian (under eye) and it quickly resolved the issue. Excited, Mary ran to a water fountain and splashed water on her face. The water phobia and nightmares disappeared and never returned. Callahan later taught his technique "Thought Field Therapy" (TFT) to those who were interested.

EFT Born: 1995

Gary Craig, a Stanford engineer and NLP Master, took the TFT training from Roger Callahan, expanded and simplified the process and evolved it into what we know today as "Emotional Freedom Techniques" (EFT).

GEMT Approach: 2011

In preparing to teach traditional EFT in 2011 at the Palo Alto School of Hypno- therapy, Robert Ranche and Dorthy Tyo studied Gary Craig's certification videos and noted that his sessions were more successful when he created rapport with the client. This led them to create "Guided Empathy Meridian Tapping" (GEMT), which combines empathetic rapport-building with self-responsibility. They introduced the idea "nothing would exist unless it had value" to combat the sense of victimhood about an ailment, knowing that most people would more readily take responsibility for something of value. They also incorporated tactile bilateral stimulation by alternating the tapping on the same meridian point on both sides of the body using both hands, which activates both hemispheres of the brain. As hypnotherapists, they set out to achieve the same shift in perception as in hypnotherapy, reversing a decision held in the subconscious. GEMT is based on the principle that "negative emotions are stored as disruptions in the body's energy system."

Quiz – Part 2

1) What type of people are we influenced by most?
   a) People we like and admire.
   b) Experts who know the most about a topic.
   c) People who understand us.
   d) Successful people who want to show us the way.

2) You realize you feel emotionally neutral about a client's situation or disease. What can you do to minimize the risk of harming the client?
   a) Nothing because you are not judging it as good or bad.
   b) Take the stance that there must be a major upside, but it is currently beyond compression.
   c) Coddle the client with extra kindness.
   d) Show sympathy to the client for experiencing that situation or disease.

3) What have desensitization techniques brought to cognitive healing modalities?
   a) Give temporary relief of fears, phobias and painful memories so they can be confronted with minimal discomfort.
   b) Permanently remove negative emotions stored in the body's energy.
   c) Cure many diseases within minutes.
   d) Make it possible to forgive someone by tapping on the forgiveness meridian.

4) Your client is overreacting while sharing a story about an interaction with another person. What is your best response?
   a) Dismiss her reaction and try to show her your elevated perspective of the issue.
   b) This is the ideal time to teach empathy to your client.
   c) Remind the client there are many ways to perceive an issue.
   d) Completely agree with her response and feelings about the situation.

5) Which is the most ideal way to perceive a client?
    a) Someone in need of your help to solve her problems.
    b) Someone who is a part of you and everything.
    c) Someone with a disease you are confident you can get rid of.
    d) Another person who will validate how great of a healer you are.

PART 3 – The GEMT Practitioner

"Leadership is about empathy. It is about having the ability to relate to and connect with people for the purpose of inspiring and empowering their lives." — Oprah Winfrey

Courage and the Practitioner

Courage is to empathetically "jump in" when you don't know where it's going to go, and you're not sure what to say next, but you trust the process enough to move forward with the session anyway. Interview conversations may produce painful memories and habitual negative thinking, and there may be normal and obvious defensiveness. When you are at ease with the client's issue, she will feel it and become more at ease. Though some practitioners may worry about energetic negative influences during a session, because we are consistently empathetically focused on finding value, negativity cannot exist unless you are in judgement.

Some GEMT practitioners will not have the opportunity to leverage their skills from other modalities, such as talk therapy and forgiveness work. GEMT attempts to start the session as quickly as possible rather than having the client talk through her issues. The concepts of forgiveness work, though they may be useful in other contexts, still portray the client as a victim. Many analysts are brilliant in their problem-solving skills; however, in GEMT there are no problems to solve. The GEMT approach to healing is for both experienced and inexperienced healing practitioners. Almost anyone who believes with certainty that nothing would exist unless it had value can be an excellent GEMT practitioner.

GEMT is a *healing art* form. In this book and course, you will learn a number of techniques that will alleviate or eliminate the pain, defensiveness, and negative thinking that accompanies or produces it. As a GEMT practitioner, you will become confident and skillful at bilateral meridian tapping, empathizing, and finding value for discomfort, ailments, and difficult situations. We invite you to consciously make the decision and commitment to become that person. This is a skills-based training, and we learn and become proficient by doing.

When to Use GEMT

GEMT can be done almost anytime, anywhere, though like all modalities, it has its place and limitations. Though it can be challenging for some clients to fully participate in the tapping and empathetic bond the first time, even the most reluctant clients will adapt to the process once emotional anesthesia sets in. The following items will help you decide if GEMT is a good choice:

- You and the client are free of distractions, i.e., people, phones, pets.
- You can hear each other clearly.
- The client is ready, willing and able to participate in a conversation.
- The client is willing to teach you what it is like to experience her issue.
- The client is comfortable with at least one of the two basic forms of teaching
  - The client leading the conversation in a way that you can repeat
  - The client allowing you to lead, correcting your assumptions when needed
- The client is comfortable with the idea of the practitioner using "I" statements and mirroring and matching while tapping on the meridian points.

The ideal client has either been a GEMT client before or is curious about trying a meridian tapping cognitive therapy, willing to participate in an Empathetic Bond, and has a strong desire to heal. Clients with previous EFT experience have the skill and knowledge of tapping on the meridian points, though sometimes slow down because they are confused by the absence of "Even though…" statements.

Clients who do personal growth work can experience more rapid healing with ease; however, they might be confused about forgiveness which might present itself with statements such as "I forgave her already. I thought I was done with that issue." A possible response could be: "And you did forgive her, without question. It's just that your subconscious somehow didn't get the message the way you intended. One way to help your subconscious interpret your intention correctly is to "thank" that (pain, person, situation, event, etc.); look what you have accomplished because of it."

Challenging Work with Great Reward

Essentially, the GEMT practitioner is required to change her perceptions and beliefs from what is "wrong" to what is "right," or from what is "bad" to what is "good." Some situations can make it difficult for a GEMT practitioner to be empathetic, e.g., a client has a history of choosing abusive relationships, and the GEMT practitioner sees the "why" or the value in the client's (as a 7-year-old) decision to equate love with abuse because the only time she was touched or given attention was when the parent abused her as a child. It is the practitioner's responsibility to come up with positive values for ailments that the client sees as negative. Using empathy, however, presents the opportunity for miraculous healing and even forgiveness with astonishing speed.

Dorthy's client Ms. S
In January 2017 a woman with weight issues became my client because "nothing she was doing, or had done, was making a difference in her food intake, her exercise, her obesity, or her disappointment with the results of all the programs she had started." As a psychotherapist who helped many other people deal with their issues, she was at a loss as to why she continued to sabotage her own health and wellness and said the one thing she had never tried was hypnosis, though she doubted she could be hypnotized.

Because she lived on the East Coast and I was located in California, our meetings were held online through video conferencing and during our first two sessions, I utilized hypnosis. She not only discovered she could be hypnotized; she also discovered the value of changing her perceptions of herself.

During our third appointment I introduced GEMT and shortly into the session she discovered that the emotions she had been holding deep in her subconscious for decades had not been dealt with at the subconscious level at all.

As she continued to empathetically follow the GEMT conversation, she ultimately discovered that identifying those emotions, valuing their existence and utilizing gratitude for them and others involved produced a "shift" deep within her; she also discovered the empowering factor of self-responsibility for past experiences and said she valued her new perception of herself as "Creator."

When the GEMT part of the session was complete I applied hypnosis, anchoring the empowering aspects and suggestions from details derived from our GEMT conversation.

No longer controlled by her subconscious beliefs and influences, she began taking care of herself in a very healthy way, and a year later she reported having reduced her weight by 70 pounds. She continued to reduce and now maintains a healthy weight and lifestyle. (It is apparent to me that she accepted the role of Creator and applied it in a powerfully beneficial way. —Dorthy Tyo)

The Purpose of a GEMT Practitioner

A healer out in the world quickly realizes that there are three types of people with dis-ease: those who are ready or open to be healed, those who can be motivated to be ready to be healed, and those who do not want to be healed. Though most individuals want some relief, not all are open to the idea of healing and, in some cases, are not fully aware of their dis-ease. There are some who do not perceive themselves as victims because they are experiencing benefits from their ailment and any offer to help them would be introducing judgment. It is also important to be aware that a practitioner's attention can have the adverse effect of prolonging or worsening the victim mentality or self-destructive behavior of those not ready to heal when the purpose of their dis-ease is to attract attention. Because of the cognitive participation process of GEMT, we highly recommend working with clients who are self-motivated, ready and open to the healing process.

The fundamental reason clients might reach out for help is that they are unconsciously in resistance to the existence of the issue they created, not necessarily to make the discomfort or ailment go away entirely. The purpose of a GEMT session is to guide the client to be at ease with the issue for which she is seeking help, not to undo or fix it. When the practitioner is at easy with the issue, the client will be at ease. Nothing would exist unless it had value, and pain and dis-ease are no exceptions. We don't get rid of anything with value; instead, we find the reason for its existence. Once the value of the dis-ease is understood, the client can choose to diminish the discomfort from the ailment. If there is no longer a need for the ailment, it will not be in the client's future experience.

Essentially, clients seek help because they feel they are a "victim of their ailment." GEMT empowers them by showing they are not victims by overturning the point of their life where they felt most victimized, typically at a difficult time in early childhood. When the client accepts that she was not a victim during that difficult time, she feels empowered to heal herself now, if she so chooses. When we are in a state of ease and self-responsibility with what we have created, we have the greatest opportunity for self-healing. During or at the end of the session, the original ailment, the discomfort, and the people of the past who were blamed for the challenging event, are thanked for helping create the opportunity for healing and growth.

Practitioner Mindfulness

The practitioner mindfully and continuously chooses her thoughts and emotions to prevent any negativity from entering the sacred space of the session. Subtle negative thinking can go unnoticed by the conscious mind especially when it is a habit. Keeping a positive attitude and looking for the upside is the most efficient way to avoid negativity. When the practitioner is at ease with the client and her issue, the client will sense it and relax.

Points for a practitioner to keep in mind:

- Allow ease by accepting the client and her situation.
- See that everything is as it should be so there is nothing to judge.
- Focus on the source of the issue instead of removing symptoms.
- Empower the client to solve her own issues by seeing them differently.
- Allow the session to provide what is best for the client.

Medical Knowledge

Having basic knowledge about a client's ailment, and any medication they might be taking, is certainly helpful prior to the start of a session. If the client feels you understand her medical condition, it could put her more at ease and help build rapport. Other than that, any knowledge beyond the basics about a client's dis-ease is not required. In GEMT all physical ailments are converted into emotional discomforts, so knowledge beyond a basic understanding of the ailment is not necessary.

The GEMT Practitioner Principles

- The client is always the creator, never the victim.
- Nothing would exist unless it had value, and the discomfort and/or ailment is no exception.
- All dis-ease has an emotional element to it.
- Emotional elements of an issue originate during a difficult situation long ago, prior to the client's ability to reason and process it.
- The ailment provides the link to healing by providing a link to the past event.
- What was perceived as a difficult time for the client as a victim in the past is actually an important element for growth for the client of today.
- The value of the difficult situation is so great it's beyond comprehension.
- The dis-ease is appreciated for bringing conscious awareness of the misperception of victimhood.

When we find value in both past and present issues, a resulting shift occurs for both issues, from the dis-ease of victimhood to the well-being of self-responsibility. When we add positive suggestions, a continuing momentum for self-empowerment increases.

Making Sure You Are Right for the Client

It is important to remember the first rule in healing is to do no harm. If you see your client's issue as problematic, you are in resistance to what is, because the issue did not spontaneously manifest; it is a product of the unchangeable past. In this resistance you are not right for the client and you should refer her to another practitioner. Continuing to work with this client risks adding to her dis-ease, rather than adding to her ease.

Signs that you are not right for the client:
- Unable to empathize with the client's situation
- Unable to explain the client's opinion and perspective back to them
- Unable to make the client feel normal or at ease

- Too negative to find positive words for a great healing opportunity
- Having resistance to what is and what has been created
- Having difficulty seeing the upside to the client's situation
- Seeing a problem instead of an opportunity
- Seeing the client as powerless or weak
- Seeing the client as a victim rather than the creator of the situation
- Seeing aspects of the situation as bad
- Thinking that abnormalities need to change or be fixed
- Seeing anything about the client's situation as wrong or a mistake
- Disagreeing with the client's past or present choices
- Disagreeing with the client's reasoning or beliefs
- Unable to find value in the client's ailment
- Cannot argue pros and cons to overturn a previous subconscious choice
- Having a goal for the session
- Disagreeing with the client's feelings
- Feeling bad when addressing the client's issue
- Analyzing instead of empathizing with the client
- Attempting to teach or be smarter than the client

To avoid hurting your client, end the session if you have any of the above signs. When you are at ease with the client and her issue, she will be at ease. Because most people dislike perceiving themselves as a victim, she will feel better as you guide her to self-responsibility. The client is never a victim, and nothing would exist unless it has value. A simple way to remember: If you are in resistance to what is, you are in dis-ease.

Discussions with New or Potential Clients

Many clients struggle a long time with their disease before reaching out for help, and their failed attempts at combating their symptoms and discomforts have only strengthened their belief in being a victim. There exists a potentially volatile situation prior to a session such that any mention of them being the creator of their illness or discomfort could cause significant resistance and adverse reactions.

It is the goal of the session for clients to make this discovery themselves because overcoming victimhood cannot be taught. This is why it is best to err on the conservative side in regard to how clients identify themselves as victims and avoid the topic entirely when outside the session.

Once a GEMT session starts, neither practitioner nor client can know where the conversation will go. It may even include the ideas of past lives or karma, which most clients believe and accept. For those who do not, or for whom it is contrary to their religion, these ideas can still be beneficial to them in a session. Either way, we avoid talking about past lives and karma prior to a session.

Some reasons why a practitioner should not ask about a client's belief in past lives:

- If she does not believe in past lives or it is against her religion, the question may increase defensiveness and decrease rapport.
- When there is a possibility that the session might go in the direction of past lives regardless of her answer, the question carries an unnecessary risk of losing trust and rapport.
- It can limit the potential healing if she prohibits the use of past lives.
- If she does believe in past lives, by bringing it up you are already steering the conversation prior to the session.

Some clients may take a proactive approach to have a connection with their practitioner by asking if she has any personal experience with similar ailments or symptoms. Though this is a positive action, it may be a subtle request for sympathy rather than empathy. When a practitioner shares sympathetic personal stories of struggles with ailments, it risks increasing dis-ease as well as takes the focus away from the client. As a general rule for all therapy, it is not appropriate for a practitioner to share personal information.

It is always a good idea to remind the client to not use drugs or alcohol prior to a session. If the client is a habitual user of drugs or alcohol, she must be clean and sober for at least 72 hours prior to a session. If the client is not a habitual user, we recommend at least 24 hours and up to 72 hours prior to a session on a case-by-case basis.

Questions and Statements When Not in Empathetic Bond

In everyday life we know that there are risks in asking personal questions. Our "friend or foe" discernment is activated when we receive a personal question that does not seem to be in alignment with the conversation and/or our relationship with the questioner. Any question beyond "How are you today?" risks a defensive response. Whether in everyday life or in a GEMT session, it is important to note that there are such things as bad inappropriate questions.

It is part of the GEMT session to make personal statements and ask questions of yourself while in Empathetic Bond such as "Why do I have this disease?" or "I know I created it for good reason." These can be very fruitful but note the "I." The important point we are making is that the use or implied use of the word "you" has an accusatory characteristic and can trigger a negative reaction in the client.

Questions out of Empathetic Bond are meant to clarify understanding, not to analyze, label, judge or bully the client. Answers to questions such as "What feelings are coming up?" and "What situations are you remembering?" are key to finding the core issue. In regression, questions such as "What is happening" and "Who is there?" are unavoidable and important in helping you understand as well as helping the client articulate the situation.

It is imperative to not make statements in any form of "You created this," for it can be perceived as an assault. Even with a positive twist, the idea of accusing a person struggling with her issue that she is causing her own suffering can be harmful. It is also important to refrain from asking closed, interrogative or combative questions such as "What is the value of your ailment?" or "How is your ailment serving you?" These types of questions can create defensiveness in the client and either prompt an incorrect answer such as "it's not," or correct rhetorical responses such as "I don't know" or "if I knew I would not be seeking help." The ailment is obviously serving the client or else it would not exist, and it is the responsibility of the practitioner to find and offer value for the ailment. Asking unfriendly or badgering questions where the most comfortable or correct response is a form of "I don't know" can add to the client's discomfort, which diminishes rapport. Clients are typically more focused on relief even when it may not be in the best interest of their healing. Even a seemingly helpful question like "What would you like to have happen?" would invariably solicit a response to remove, fix, or modify a symptom and bypass why it might be valuable. However, questions like "What would you like to work on?" or "What is bothering you today?" set a starting point where the symptom can be viewed as valuable.

When to Refer a Client

There are conscious and unconscious reasons why a client is drawn to a particular practitioner in regard to her chances of success. The effort put into researching, deciding, and taking the initiative to set up an appointment has started a healing momentum with a particular practitioner in mind. It is in the best interest of the client to take this into consideration prior to referring her to another practitioner.

There is certainly enough reason to refer a client if you are in judgment about her particular ailment. However, this might be a motivating opportunity to do personal healing prior to the session. Instead of immediately referring to a client who has an ailment you have a negative association with, attempt to have an imaginary session where the ailment is viewed as a perfect metaphor to change a negative perspective. If possible, use bilateral tapping while visualizing someone you know with the ailment as the client. If you are successful in changing your view on the ailment, your client will benefit as well.

If you still feel you are not right for a particular client, validate the client for selecting you anyway. Your referral can add to her healing momentum by her feeling she is on the right path. Avoid sharing details on whether the practitioner has previous experience with her ailment, so she does not have sympathetic expectations. Give an intuitive reason why this particular practitioner can help her so that she can continue to open to the possibility of healing.

Mission Statement for the Professional GEMT Practitioner

Writing a mission statement can be helpful to future clients and to you as a practitioner.

Some of the benefits of a GEMT Mission Statement

- Helping differentiate your healing practice from others.
- Communicating your strengths to potential clients.
- Helping prepare clients for what to expect in a session.
- Helping you focus on what you believe is important in healing.

An example of a GEMT Mission Statement:

I am from the school of thought that your true identity is that of a perfect and pure loving being. I respect what you value, without judgment, and I understand that we keep what we value. I know that many times the memories and decisions we value are stored as painful disruptions in our body's energy system. I am very curious about your suffering and will use guided empathy to walk with you while you heal yourself. So we can deeply explore your suffering, we will use bilateral meridian tapping as an emotional anesthesia to help reduce pain and defensiveness. I believe that healing is a "change in perception." During our GEMT session, you will have the opportunity to shift your perception of old wounds and hidden traumas and transform your issue.

Your Mission Statement:

Quiz - Part 3

1) Excellent GEMT practitioners are
   a) Almost anyone who believes with certainty that nothing would exist unless it had value.
   b) Practitioners who are adept at forgiveness work.
   c) Therapists experienced in allowing their clients to talk through their issues.
   d) Analysts who have an innate ability for problem solving.

2) You have just facilitated a GEMT session where the client ultimately resolved her chronic pain which has kept her in a wheelchair for years. While in a department store, you see a man in a wheelchair and, feeling confident from the session earlier, have the urge to approach him to offer your help healing his ailment. How would this be inappropriate and potentially harmful to him?
   a) You have specific wants about a session with him.
   b) You do not know whether his ailment is fueled by attention given to it.
   c) You are assuming he perceives himself as a victim.
   d) All the above.

3) You have a new client who wants to see you for arthritis which reminds you of your aunt's painful bout with the disease. What is best to do before the session?
   a) Immediately refer the client to another practitioner who does not have a prejudice with the disease.
   b) Have an imaginary session with your aunt where the arthritis is viewed as an enormously valuable and perfect symptom for her realization of a new perspective and healing something in her life.
   c) Understand as much as you can about the disease.
   d) Prepare to share your sympathetic stories about your aunt's struggles.

4) A new client calls to make an appointment with you for a chronic disease she feels that she has had since birth. Because symptoms seem to come and go at random, she feels the ailment is controlling her life. While on the phone with her, what aspect(s) of the session should you discuss?
   a) Ask her whether or not she believes in past lives.
   b) Inform her that the session will be about her realizing she has been the creator of her ailment all along.
   c) Refrain from drugs and alcohol before the session.
   d) All the above.

5) Which question(s) is/are helpful when not in an Empathetic Bond?
   a) "What would you like to have happen?"
   b) "How is your ailment serving you?"
   c) "What situations are you remembering?"
   d) All the above

PART 4 – How To Do GEMT

"That which we persist in doing becomes easier for us to do; not that the nature of the thing itself is changed, but that our power to do it is increased." — Ralph Waldo Emerson

The Step-by-Step Process of a GEMT Session

These steps are general guidelines to help you keep the flow of the session when first learning GEMT. Steps 1 through 5 and 12 through 14 are consistently used. However, as you become more experienced, we encourage you to modify, add, bypass or repeat any of the other steps when it suits a particular session. GEMT sessions are conversations about utilizing current issues as beacons to reveal and overturn old misperceptions of victimhood. A natural easy conversation is best (see Appendix for examples of actual sessions).

1. Say the client's name, then raise the client's vibration.
2. Get the starting-point issue with details (What, When, and SUDS).
3. Start tapping three complete rounds while explaining GEMT and tapping.
4. Start Empathetic Bond. Have the client repeat, gently, "So, I have this _____ issue...."
5. Say what you know about the issue (What, When, and SUDS).
6. State assumptions about having the issue; the client will correct you.
7. Continue building trust with the client's subconscious, while learning about the disease.
    a. When the client leads or corrects, make sure to repeat and follow closely and accurately as possible using the client's choice of words.
    b. Offer contrasting thoughts when the client is unsure of the answer.

8. Define the emotion about the issue.
   a. Something about the ailment, pain or situation does not seem fair. Qualify the unfairness as an emotion (fear, anger, resentment, sadness, etc.)
   b. Explain that all discomforts have a particular and unique emotional element without exception.
9. Take the client back to the source issue by suggesting that the emotion is familiar to a difficult situation long ago by an analogy such as
   a. "I am not having a reasonable emotional response for this issue. It is because the situation is just reminding me of a similar situation long ago. Before I had reasoning skills. When I was a child."
   b. "Like a familiar song from long ago, I remember when I first had this emotion."
10. Address feelings of victimhood, then plant the seed of responsibility.
   a. Suggest that in that difficult situation she perceived herself as a victim.
   b. Then, present the perspective that we are never a victim of something of value and/or offer pros and uncertainty.
   c. Then, empower the client with "Why would I put myself through this?"
11. Offer a plausible beneficial scenario as to why the event might be chosen.
   a. Use your imagination to tell a metaphoric story that gives value to the difficult event that your client (or client's subconscious) will accept.
   b. E.g., Strength for later in life, being free of subconscious guilt, etc.
   c. "You chose it because you knew you could handle it."
12. Thank the people who were part of the difficult situation and helped the lessons be learned, karma be paid, goal be accomplished, etc.
13. Thank the pain and/or ailment that brought the opportunity for great healing.
14. Stop tapping and get the starting point issue SUDS.
15. Use hypnotherapy to expedite the healing and close the session.

Note-taking with GEMT

Because the original issue is viewed as an alert to look at something bigger, in-depth interview questions or notes are not needed or recommended because it is not the focus of the session. Pausing your focus on the client to take notes could hinder the building of rapport and potentially create a feeling in the client of being analyzed. Note-taking is also a disruption in the conversation, and it creates unequal roles, which can slow the achievement of trust needed for the Empathetic Bond. We recommend those who want to keep records and notes about their sessions record the session audibly and make notes post-session.

GEMT Session Structure (In Person)

- Quiet room with few distractions
- Similar chairs / Sitting upright / Facing each other
- Knee distance approximately 12 inches (30 centimeters)

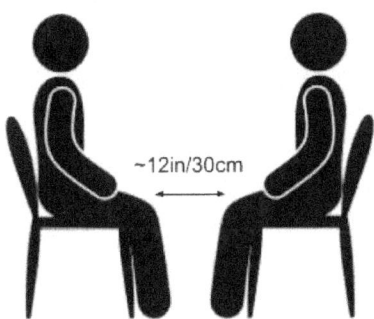

~12in/30cm

Analogies for Explaining the Subconscious Mind

1.   The subconscious mind is like deep fertile soil that accepts any seed you plant within it. Habitual thoughts and beliefs are seeds that are being constantly planted within and produce in your life/body what is sown. As surely as tomato seeds produce tomatoes and wheat seeds produce wheat, thoughts produce an effect in one's life. You will reap what you sow. This is the law of cause and effect. With the conscious mind as the gardener, it is our responsibility to be aware of how this process works, and to choose

wisely what we are planting. Rarely was our role as gardener ever explained to us, and we have allowed seeds of all types, both good and bad, to enter the garden of our subconscious. These "seeds of thought" manifest success, abundance and health as easily as failure, ill health and challenges. Our subconscious accepts the thoughts (seeds) sown with emotions and repetition, whether these thoughts are positive or negative, and does not evaluate things the way the conscious mind does.

2.   The subconscious mind is simply a tool that we have not been taught how to use effectively. An analogy often used is that "the human brain is the most powerful supercomputer on the planet; we just never got the user manual." Without the "user manual" our minds run rampant, with limited knowledge of how to correct the issues that were created by a lack of understanding. When we perceive the subconscious mind as a tool rather than an entity with good or bad intentions or some "master plan" to direct our lives, we can begin to understand how to use it to our benefit. It works like a storage unit, similar to a hard drive on a computer. Information is collected through our various senses and simply stored. Another similarity is that, like a computer, when the information is stored in the subconscious mind, it is "indexed" so that when our conscious mind needs specific information, there is a way to retrieve it.

3.   The subconscious operates like a modern-day computer but has a storage capacity and memory system that surpasses ordinary computers by petabytes beyond comprehension. The subconscious mind is a personal computer, and YOU are the computer's operator. It records everything that happens in the personal, sensory and intellectual world—from the day of conception until the day of death. It takes directions from the perceptions of the conscious mind and follows these directions implicitly. It might be called the world's most obedient servant. It can only say "yes." It has no limitations. It has no past and no future; it functions only in present tense. Every thought becomes part of the never-failing memory system of the subconscious mind. EACH INDIVIDUAL IS WHAT HE THINKS. When we understand that our thoughts create and shape our reality, we will be more careful and selective with our choice of thoughts.

80

Raising the Client's Vibration and Getting the Starting Point Issue

Raising our vibration (mood) also raises our consciousness and causes us to think differently. Here is an example of raising the client's vibration and then asking what they would like to work on, and you may have your own techniques as well.

Relax, take an easy inhale, a relaxing exhale, and gently close your eyes. Imagine a pure loving white light is entering through the top of your head and filling every cell in your body with loving vibration. Imagine you are surrounded by the people of the past, present, and future who love you. Imagine every good deed you have ever done has been brought into the present moment. Now multiply that feeling times infinity. That is who you really are. Take an easy inhale, a gentle exhale, and open your eyes when you are ready. What would you like to work on today?

The response will be used later to start the conversation. Here is an example of getting the starting point issue details with possible answers in parentheses:

1. What would you like to work on today? ("My anxiety.")
2. Describe how it feels. ("It feels very shaky inside me.")
3. What is the discomfort on a scale from 0 to 10? ("About an 8.")
4. When did it first start? ("Three years ago.")
5. What was happening around the time it started? ("I was fired from my job.")
6. Who was involved? ("The manager.")

The details are the first words shared in Empathetic Bond after the opening statement of "So, I have this anxiety issue, yet nothing would exist unless it had value, and this anxiety (that is shaky inside me) that is an 8 and started about 3 years ago because my manager fired me, is no exception." This is a free-flowing conversation.

Qualifying Issues

One of the distinguishing facets of GEMT is the way it qualifies dis-ease. Because every issue or ailment is viewed as a great opportunity for deep healing, the practitioner qualifies it as a good, or even a great, manifestation. Every session starts by the practitioner qualifying the client's starting point issue. This sets the tone for the whole session and helps the client follow the practitioner in her curiosity as to why her ailment is so great. Ailments are rich in metaphor, brilliantly symbolic of misperceptions and create social synchronicities for the opportunity to heal existing relationships and/or create new ones. Issues can also be qualified as they come up in a session, which can add to the certainty of being on the path to great healing. Use common sense and practicality by qualifying issues enough to raise the vibration and curiosity of the client while maintaining sincerity.

Immediately after qualifying the issue, continue asking for details which gives the qualification a subliminal effect of raising the client's vibration and lightening the mood of the session. It is important to not linger after qualifying an issue to maintain its subtle but powerful effect on preparing the client for deep healing.

Examples of qualifying an issue and immediately getting starting point details:

- Client: "My anxiety is at 10 when I have to speak in public."
  Practitioner: "That's fantastic. How often do you have to speak in public?"

- Client: "I have had this back pain since I was laid off."
  Practitioner: "That's great. Have you ever had a similar back pain?"

- Client: "I have this out-of-control skin disease."
  Practitioner: "That's amazing. When did you first notice it?"

Qualifying an issue is analogous to giving someone genuine praise for her novice paintings, and your appreciation beyond the intrinsic value allows her to feel a deeper sense of acceptance and rapport with you. Issues become a celebration of personal expression and ability to create. Failure to qualify her issue as a good thing risks her assuming that you agree with her perception that it is bad. Qualifying an issue as good at the start of the session sets a positive tone that health and wellness are certain.

Start Tapping

It is important to start the tapping process as soon as possible to help keep the healing momentum going after the starting point issue is found. Delaying the tapping to talk more about the issue can lower the client's vibration and even cause the starting point issue to change. Once the starting point issue is found and the SUDS established, the "sharing of details" portion of the session is over. If the client wants to talk more about her issue at this time, explain that it is best to begin tapping while continuing the conversation and see where things go. You can say something like "Let's jump in. It's best to tell me more while we tap and see where things go." It is key to the rapport building technique of mirroring that both client and practitioner are tapping on their same respective points as much as possible.

Explaining GEMT to a Client

After the client has learned the tapping points and knows to follow you, GEMT is explained while continuing to tap. Avoid ideas about overturning victimhood, past lives, and karma. Allow it to be implied that she is expected to participate by tapping, repeating, and correcting. For example,

GEMT is like having a regular everyday conversation while we are also tapping on meridian points; the same meridian points used in acupuncture and acupressure. We tap on these points so we can have a conversation about anything without getting defensive. For example, if I said, "That wall is purple" and you were not tapping you might say, "Hey, it's not purple; you are trying to trick me." But if you were tapping you would calmly say, "No it's not." The purpose is not to problem solve but for me to understand what it is like to have ___ so you can see it in me. Because its often easier to heal someone else than it is to heal ourself. To help me understand your perspective, we will both repeat each other using "I" statements, and please correct me when my assumptions are not true. Feel free to lead the conversation when you discover something. Ok, I will start.

Use Your Own Style Guiding the Client

Though a GEMT session is a flow of consciousness and can go any which way depending on the responses from the client, you have the opportunity to develop your own style and share higher perspectives about well-being. Higher perspectives might include ideas from *A Course In Miracles*, Abraham-Hicks, St. Germain, Buddha, and many others.

For example, while tapping in empathetic bond, you might guide with

"It seems like I am in a difficult situation at my job, yet I have the power to move mountains."

The client will usually accept and repeat the statement while tapping in empathetic bond, and the studies of Applied Kinesiology show us such a statement will "muscle test" as true. When the client is not tapping, ego defenses often reject such a statement. In a GEMT session, regularly offer empowering positive perspectives for the client to handle her current situation to bring ease and gain clarity on the negative emotion.

GEMT Session Conversation

A GEMT session is simply a conversation with the added purpose of attempting to understand what it is like to experience what the client is experiencing (to walk a mile in the client's moccasins.) This process brings two new key perspectives. One, you can share a new perspective about the issue, and two, the client gains the perspective of seeing her issue in someone else. It is important to not assume in any way that you know what the issue is or where the conversation is going to go.

When first learning GEMT, the practitioner can sometimes feel stuck, not knowing where to guide the conversation. This is most likely because the practitioner has forgotten the steps or some of the philosophical concepts. It is not ideal for the client to suspect you are stuck by you awkwardly pausing the session or for you to verbally disclose it to her. The ideal way to handle a situation when you are stuck is to understand where you are and where you want to go next based on the philosophical concepts. The session always goes forward, never backward.

GEMT basic flow outline:
1. **Convert the physical ailment to an emotion.**
   a. Whether physical or emotional, GEMT treats all ailments as emotional dis-ease.
   b. Once converted, physical aspects will not be discussed until the end of the session.
   c. Offer contrasting thoughts if needed
2. **Uncover a childhood traumatic event with a similar emotion.**
   a. The emotion of a current disease is often caused by an overreaction learned in childhood prior to the development of reasoning skills.
   b. Once the childhood issue is found the emotion of the current disease is no longer discussed.
3. **Confront the core issue.**
   a. Validate feelings and reactions as normal and understandable.
   b. Offer pros and uncertainty if needed.
4. **Plant the seed of responsibility.**
   a. "Why would I put myself through this?"
   b. Once the seed of responsibility is planted, childhood reactions and feelings are no longer discussed.
5. **Offer/suggest enormous value for the core event.**
   a. Personal growth, resolve karma, resolve past life trauma, etc.
   b. Offering value helps the client take responsibility for the event, especially now that the mission is accomplished, lessons have been learned, the karma has been paid, etc.

6. **Once the client accepts responsibility, thank the ailment and people involved.**
   a. When the purpose of the ailment is realized, it can be released.
   b. We are not victims when we thank instead of forgiving.
7. **Check in with the original issue.**
   a. Compare SUDS and discomfort to values before the session.
   b. Quantifying success strengthens the client and the healing process.

Once you understand the philosophical basis of GEMT and with adequate practice, you will have a better understanding of what to say.

The practitioner leads the beginning of the session, and often the entire session. When leading, the practitioner makes assumptions about the client's situation and encourages the client to correct her. Incorrect assumptions are inevitable and even deliberate at times, so there is never a need to apologize. It is, however, important for the practitioner to repeat verbatim the client's corrections with "I" statements to maintain the empathetic bond and increase rapport. Intentionally making an incorrect assumption to demonstrate that the practitioner will say what the client says is one of the subtle ways to increase rapport and encourage the client to lead. As the client corrects, she is now leading the session, and the amount of time a client leads can vary greatly. Be mindful to pick up the lead when the client seems finished leading, so the flow continues. Pausing the session during a correction risks losing rapport. Client corrections are a valuable and critical time in the session.

There is often "stalling" by the practitioner to gain more emotional anesthesia from tapping, and a weaving back and forth to gently prepare the client for possibly the most difficult concept to hear: that she is the creator and not the victim of her difficult situations. It is your responsibility to come up with the value ideas for her ailment. She will follow you in her curiosity of why you think her ailment is great.

Remember that your role as a GEMT practitioner is to empathetically understand what it is like to have the client's issue, and to not judge her perceptions as needing correction. The only misperception GEMT focuses on is that of victimhood. When your client no longer perceives herself as a victim, additional empowerment comes as she self-corrects misperceptions. You would be doing your client a disservice by persuading her to correct them prior to that time.

Assumptions about a client's situation:

- The client's current painful emotional reaction is a re-stimulation of an early childhood traumatic event that happened prior to the age of eight.
- The client is never a victim, always the creator, i.e., she created the early childhood traumatic event.
- The early childhood traumatic event has value and was created for a reason that is more than worth the suffering that has occurred from it.

What if the Client Does Not Follow the Practitioner's Tapping?

Clients occasionally become distracted by their thoughts and neglect to follow the practitioner to the next tapping point. When this occurs, go back to the tapping point the client is on and treat it as a new point by tapping on it seven to nine times. Then, with eye contact, make a more obvious movement to the next tapping point. If you feel it necessary, call out the name of the tapping point (e.g., "side-of-eye"). If the client still does not follow you in cycling through the tapping points or stops tapping all together, pause the session and discuss whether or not to continue with this modality.

What if the Client Stops Repeating?

If the client stops repeating while in an empathetic bond, try contrasting thoughts instead of repeating the statement or going down a different path.

Repeating the same statement risks increasing dis-ease and losing rapport if the client perceives that as an attempt to persuade her to accept your agenda. Keep the momentum of the conversation going rather than pausing, stalling or waiting until the client repeats. It is often an indication that you are on the right path when the client is not repeating your statements.

Common Phrases in a GEMT Session

a) "Nothing would exist unless it had value, and this _____ is no exception."

b) "All ailments/issues have an emotional element, and this _____ is no exception."

c) "There is an aspect about this _____ that seems unfair which stirs my emotions."

d) "And the emotional aspect of this particular issue is _____" (pause to allow the client to answer with an emotional aspect, word or phrase, such as anger, hatred, sadness, frustration, guilt)

e) "Part of me would like to say I invented this particular _____, yet it is pretty common to have this as a result of my life experience."

f) "Anyone would have this _____ (emotional aspect) if they were in my shoes in that situation."

g) "I am glad I have this _____ (emotional aspect) because it means I care and helps me to have greater clarity about what I do want."

h) "All reactions are learned, and I was overreacting in that situation. When and where did I learn that reaction?"

i) "Like emotions felt from hearing a familiar song from years ago, I can remember when I first had this particular emotional issue."

j) "I am not having this emotional response for the reason I think I do. The situation is just reminding me of a similar situation long ago. Before I had reasoning skills. When I was a child."

k) "Someone did not meet my expectations. I think I know who."

l) "If I had to choose between feeling criticized or disliked, I would choose _____."

m) "The value of the difficult situation is beyond my comprehension, and it has allowed me to ____."

n) "I am actually grateful for this _____ situation, because it prepared me perfectly for later in life, and that is why it is coming up now."

o) "I want to thank my original _____ issue, for letting me know that I was ready to resolve a much bigger issue from my past."

p) "Because I am an enlightened old soul, with ancient wisdom, all of this makes absolute sense to me."

See Appendix for a chart of a vocabulary of feelings to utilize with people who need help identifying their feelings.

Contrasting Thoughts

Offering contrasting thoughts is optional when the session is progressing with ease, though it can help prepare for overturning homeostasis when pros and uncertainty are offered to traumatic events later in the session. However, it becomes necessary to offer contrasting thoughts when the client becomes quieter or stops repeating. This can either be because she is unsure, or some memory has come up that is distracting her. Pausing the session when the client is not repeating risks losing rapport and should only be done if you feel confident that a question like "What is coming up?" will have an answer. The best option when a client is not repeating is to first offer contrasting thoughts.

Examples of contrasting thoughts:

- I FEEL dis-ease in my body / I DO NOT FEEL dis-ease in my body.
- This ____ ailment IS a dis-ease / This _____ ailment IS NOT a dis-ease.
- I am/am not at ease in the world.
- People should/should not be able do what they want.
- My dis-ease will/won't change people's behavior.
- It feels good/bad to criticize and complain.
- I love/hate mistakes when I am learning or practicing.

- Great discoveries did/did not come from experiencing mistakes.
- People should be allowed/should not be allowed to make mistakes.
- My dis-ease will/won't stop mistakes from happening.
- I accept/reject my body.
- I chose/did not choose my body.
- I am at ease/disease with my body.
- I do/do not have the power to choose.
- I can choose to be at ease/dis-ease about the world/people/my body.
- I am at ease/dis-ease in life.
- I would rather learn than judge/judge than learn from the situation.
- It feels good/bad to learn/judge.

If a client will not repeat any of the contrasting statements you offer, pause the session and check in with the client. There might be valuable thoughts for the client to share. There is also a possibility that GEMT may not be the ideal modality for this particular client.

Pausing the Session

Pausing the session means to stop tapping, leading, and the repeating of empathetic "I" statements. Though most sessions have short pauses, the breaking of the empathetic bond risks losing rapport, momentum and emotional anesthesia. For this reason, the session should not be paused unless

- You feel a short pause with directed questions can help the client share specific details better, such as "Who is there?" and "What is happening?"
- The client is physically tired or "buzzing" from the tapping.
- The client is not repeating contrasting statements.

Stalling

In GEMT, stalling is when the practitioner deliberately slows down the session. There are a few reasons why you might want to slow down or "stall" a session:

- To encourage the client to lead.
- To allow more time for the client to process what has already occurred.
- To allow extra time to create more emotional anesthesia before continuing.

Some methods of stalling are

- Slowing down speech.
- Breaking up repeated sentences into phrases or words.
- Using "um" or other hesitation sounds.
- Using empty statements such as "and I'm not sure what happened next."

Avoid stalling when the client is not repeating because it risks losing rapport and might be perceived as belittling.

Common Mistakes to Avoid

- Using "you" instead of "I"
- Not waiting for the client to mirror your tapping point (mirroring)
- Not repeating the client verbatim (matching)
- Seeing the client as a victim of the ailment or situation
- Not tapping long enough during a session
- Not establishing SUDS (0 – 10) scale before beginning the session
- Focusing on a situation where the client is overacting rather than where the reaction was originally learned
- Focusing on symptoms rather than misperceptions

Important Points to Remember

- Help the client accept where she is right now.
- Practitioner is responsible for maintaining the conversation.
- All reactions are learned.
- Overreactions are a re-stimulation of a traumatic event.
- Give yourself poetic license to change perceptions.

Reading the Nuances of Client Feedback

When the client is confronting a difficult situation, it is important to be sensitive to and aware of the client's level of comfort. If the client seems overwhelmed by showing signs like stressful breathing, hesitation in repeating, looking down, or even tears, respond by "stalling" or backing away from the issue. It is important to continue tapping with empathetic patience to create more emotional anesthesia while the client regains composure before continuing.

Actions to take when a client is overwhelmed:

- Continue tapping and do not pause the session. Encourage the client to begin tapping again if she has stopped.
- Stay in an empathetic bond with "I" statements and do not make or imply "you" questions or statements.
- Lead with powerful affirmations and stop giving attention to the event.
- Stall by continuing to tap, slowing down words and breaking up sentences.
- Add more emotional anesthesia (side-to-side eye movement, deep breathing).

The client is either in agreement, disagreement, or unsure when following the empathetic guide of the practitioner. It is very important to be aware of signs suggesting the client is unsure. Typically, when feeling unsure, she may look away, or respond with an "uh" or "um" instead of repeating what you said, or possibly not repeat at all. If the client is showing signs of being unsure, you can offer contrasting thoughts. For example, "My father

DOES deserve my love" … (no response), then… "My father DOES NOT deserve my love" …. (no response), then again, "My father DOES deserve my love," and the client will now typically respond by repeating the last statement.

It is also important to be aware of when the client experiences a "shift" or "aha!" moment, indicating a profound change in perception. When this occurs, the client's facial features, posture and breathing can be seen as more relaxed, and sometimes she will exude a sense of confidence and self-empowerment. Though the client may want to stop tapping, it is important to encourage her to continue tapping during the transition from dis-ease to ease while instilling the new perception without defensiveness.

Defensiveness and Defusing

The client is at ease when you are at ease with the client and her issue. The opposite is also true in that a client can become defensive if she senses any judgment from you about her or her issue. Even when you are more at ease with her and her issue than she is, she can bring defensiveness from her own judgment. This is why it is imperative for you to embrace "what is" as a perfect product of the unchangeable past. Even when you convey that there is nothing wrong with her or her issue, defensiveness can be lurking in her attachment to judging past events. Your compassionate guidance is your most valuable tool to navigate defensiveness.

One way to defuse defensiveness is to approach the issue from a different direction, rather than head on. In hypnotherapy, for example, an idea may be introduced as a metaphor, which allows a less intrusive way to deal with the transformation of an issue. In GEMT, because we are in cognitive conversation, we attempt to avoid the defensiveness and resistance to change by talking around the issue first. For example, a generic statement like "There were a lot of things happening during that time in my life" can be helpful to defuse defensiveness. Once we notice that the client's defensiveness has relaxed, we can talk about the core issue with the same attitude and intensity as the casual non-issue topics. This technique also quickly provides the client with a perspective that the issue is smaller than originally perceived. From this point, deep transformation can quickly begin by looking at the issue from a new perspective.

Finding the Earliest Experience of Victimhood

Through our studies and experience using GEMT we have been able to find the source issue without too much effort, because the current issue is a re-stimulation of the source issue. This is why the current issue is so valuable, it is bringing up the memory of the core issue that is ready to be healed.

All ailments and discomfort have an emotional element of victimhood where, for example, the client either does not believe she chose the situation or had no free will to change it. The most prevalent, current issue provides the best opportunity to uncover the earliest victimhood experience. After reiterating the emotional aspects of the current issue, ask for a familiar emotion during a difficult time long ago. This will usually uncover the challenging event.

One method of finding the matching emotion is to use the reference of a familiar song from long ago. When we hear a song from decades past, emotions are triggered as if the distant memory happened yesterday.

For example, while tapping in empathetic bond, you might guide the client to repeat one of these phrases:
- "I have this _____ (emotion) from the _____ (issue), yet it is not the first time I have felt this emotion. Like a familiar song long ago, I remember when I first had this _____ feeling. I was a young child."
- "I would like to say, 'So what' about this ___ (issue) I have, but there are aspects that seem unfair. I had a similar feeling of unfairness as a child."
- "I could rationalize this situation, yet there is a strong emotion preventing me from doing that. The emotion is particular, and it is like how I felt as a child when. . ."

- "I am not sure if it's that I feel like I'm unlovable or that I'm not enough..."

Then, breaking from empathetic bond, try directly asking the client
- "What memories are coming up?"
- "How old might you be?"
- "Where could you be?"
- "What could be happening?"

The client's response reveals the earliest experience that she perceived herself as a victim. Though there may be many childhood traumas, this particular GEMT session will focus on overturning the particular event that surfaced where the client believed she was a victim. Because we are never victims of "something of value," when we find value for a traumatic event, it helps release us from victimhood.

Note: We understand that traditional therapists might see this as an antithetical viewpoint regarding childhood trauma. However, utilizing emotional anesthesia from bilateral meridian tapping allows the client to reconsider old perceptions.

Possible feelings from childhood traumas:
- Abandoned
- Ignored
- Unprotected
- Criticized
- Bullied
- Abused

Once the earliest experience of victimhood is found, there is no more blaming, assigning fault, or even forgiving. The traumatic event is to be seen in its original difficulty before planting the seed of responsibility.

Subconscious Re-evaluation by Offering Pros and Uncertainty

The subconscious interprets our misperceptions as intention and therefore manifests that intention as an ailment. For a client to be in resistance to the ailment the subconscious ultimately created for her benefit, she creates a whole new level of dis-ease for herself. This can be addressed by offering benefits, or pros, of why the ailment would exist. Offering pros not only reduces the dis-ease about having the ailment, but it also opens the subconscious to reveal the negative emotions and misperceptions that ultimately caused the ailment. In GEMT, the practitioner might be thought of as a defense attorney, viewing the client's current issue as a consequence of the best decision she could make during an extremely stressful time long ago.

Concepts and perceptions that originated during stressful situations in life are stored in the subconscious mind. Subconsciously, we make split-second decisions based on perception, habits, and beliefs created from previous experiences or decisions. The subconscious then directs the body to obediently provide the resulting condition and symptoms that the client now wants to heal.

The best way to work with the subconscious decision-making process in a GEMT session is to speak in terms of pros and cons. Using GEMT has shown that overturning a subconscious interpretation is quick and simple if both the pros and cons are addressed during the session. Because the cons are adequately represented and expressed by the suffering client, any benefit (pro) that the GEMT practitioner can present opens the subconscious for change. The subconscious processes thousands of bits of information per second more than the conscious mind, and when a previous perception is reversed or overturned quickly, a shift is felt physically as well as emotionally.

The strength of a belief correlates to the certainty of the perception upon which it is based. When uncertainty about her original perceptions is presented, the client has the opportunity to change her limiting beliefs in the session. For example, if a client believes that he is unsuccessful in life because he struck out in a baseball game at the age of 10, offer pros and uncertainty with a statement like "It was good that I struck out at that game when I was 10 years old because the pressure to succeed at that time would have been too great for me ... or not." Here the pros and uncertainty ("or not" statement) presented by the practitioner brings the original perception into question. From that point the client can make a new decision which changes his beliefs.

Examples of pros, cons and uncertainty:
- "Maybe being sent off to boarding school made me more independent ... or maybe it didn't."
- "I am glad I had an abusive father because it made me more compassionate with my own children ... or not."
- "Being abandoned as a child helps me understand other people's abandonment issues ... or it doesn't."
- "Not being allowed to express myself as a child has made me aware of the importance of self-expression ... or maybe it doesn't."
- "Having a hurt leg got me out of doing work during that time ... or maybe it didn't."
- "Having that illness as a child got me more attention than if I didn't have it ... or maybe it made no difference."
- "Being able to forgive my abusive parents has given me a deep understanding of the compassion I am capable of ... or not."

Planting the Seed of Responsibility

Once the core issue is found, there is no blaming, assigning of fault, or even forgiveness. This is the time to plant the seed of responsibility that will ultimately facilitate overturning victimhood. Pivoting from victim to creator starts with a short statement just before the value of the traumatic event is presented to the client. This subtle idea of her being the creator of her most victimhood experience is the most important statement to make while in an empathetic bond during this time.

Example statements of planting the seed of responsibility:
- "Why would I put myself through this?"
- "Why did I choose to put myself in this situation?"
- "There must be a good reason why I would put myself in this situation."

The Value of Difficult Situations

Nothing would exist unless it has value, and we are the creator of our experiences. Difficult experiences are no exception. To help the client perceive herself as the creator of the difficult event, use your intuition to find the most valuable and acceptable reason why she might choose it. Here, we list examples of the values that can be derived from difficult situations for a client:

- A lesson on values and a better understanding of what is important
- Creating a situation where a lesson is unavoidable and inescapable
- Strength for later in life
- Growth out of a limiting comfort zone
- Uncovering and healing deep-seated resentment and anger
- Development of an empathetic perspective to heal others later in life
- Learning what to do or not to do, such as in being a better parent
- Spiritual growth through not letting a bad situation define you
- Self-love—rising from the experience is what you love most about yourself
- Balancing karma from a past life of causing suffering for someone else
- Creating an opportunity to learn forgiveness from the premise "they know not what they do"
- Being of service by demonstrating or teaching how to forgive
- Agreeing to play a healing role for the abuser regardless of the actions
- Resolving or conquering a traumatic or fatal experience that happened as an adult in a previous life

Using the Idea of Past Lives

As a rule, a client will not repeat a GEMT practitioner's statement in empathetic bond if she does not believe it could be true. The one exception is when the idea of past lives is introduced. It has been demonstrated that even when a client states before a session that she does not believe in past lives, she will follow the practitioner's guiding statements about a past life if it tends to give her a logical explanation as to why a childhood issue existed. In general, it's best to avoid using the term "past life" in a session, and instead use phrases like "centuries ago," "thousands of years ago," or even simply, "long, long ago." More often than not, a client who did not believe in past lives prior to a session often expresses surprise after the session that she followed along with the idea of a past life, especially when she experienced great healing as a result.

NOTE: As a practitioner, if you are someone who doubts your ability to create a relatable "past life" scenario for your client during a session, remember Aristotle's pronouncement, "A vivid imagination compels the body to obey it." The story you offer will come to you because of what is being discovered during the tapping/conversation and *whatever that story is* will be *vividly* accepted, or not, by the client. Her subconscious mind will interpret that scenario and subsequent action of empathy and understanding as intention. This new intention causes the subconscious mind to produce healthier directives to her body, mind, emotions and behavior. It does not matter if it is an actual "past life." As she vividly accepts it consciously, literally or metaphorically, her subconscious accepts it as well.

There are at least two common uses where the idea of a past life can be helpful in a session. First, because all emotional reactions are learned, when a client feels or believes she was born with emotional distress; even before being in the womb, it often makes sense that her reaction was learned in a past life. Second, because we are always the creator of our experiences, a client will often accept the idea that a difficult childhood experience was a deliberate creation to resolve karma, or what we call "subconscious guilt."

Subconscious Guilt

It is fair to assume that most clients will be familiar with the spiritual theory of karma. The idea of karma can be a powerful tool to explain why traumatic events happened at such a young age. It also can provide value for a childhood traumatic event when viewed as freeing the client from karmic debt. Though karma can be a useful tool in a session, some spiritual teachings state that there is no karma. To avoid the term karma, we present the idea of what we call "subconscious guilt" to the client. Though it is used in reference to past lives, it's based on the common emotion of guilt. While tapping, the practitioner guides and explains that the client has already been forgiven, yet because of her own feelings of guilt, she chose to experience what it was like to be on the receiving side of her own previous careless actions. Explain that by forgiving those she blames for her traumatic childhood event, she is essentially forgiving herself of her actions from "long ago," which now frees her of subconscious guilt. Then guide the client towards the idea that the difficulty in enduring such a traumatic childhood event was more than worth it with a statement such as "that was a small price to pay to be free of that guilt." Then, guide the client into appreciation with a statement like "I would like to thank the players of my childhood traumatic event for the opportunity to free myself of subconscious guilt." This often results in a new perspective that eliminates the original issue instantly.

Bob's client Mr. P

While visiting a friend, I agreed, at her request, to help her neighbor who was suffering from back issues from an accident that occurred at his work about a year before. We held the session in the living room of my friend's house while she and her husband observed. He said he was in constant back pain, though it varied in intensity from "a 4 to an 8" and he did not like the idea of not working nor of being on disability. We started the GEMT session and reviewed how, when and why it happened and the emotion associated with the pain. The emotions identified were fear and sadness.

Exploring when he first felt this particular type of fear and sadness, he recalled being bullied by neighborhood kids at the age of six or seven because he was slower and weaker than the other kids due to a small handicap from birth. We then asked, "Why would I choose to put myself in situations of being bullied?" which transported us to "long, long ago" when he resonated with being a powerful warrior. He connected with the idea of being a Viking and brought up that he liked Viking memorabilia for some reason. I presented the idea that he bullied his Viking brothers in that lifetime who were not as strong as he was, and he has felt guilty about that, all these lifetimes. This allowed the idea that he wanted to be bullied this lifetime to feel what that was like and to finally forgive his behavior and relieve himself of guilt. He then realized that he felt he was bullied by his boss into the unsafe condition at work which caused the accident and that this all makes sense now. We recognized how perfect the handicap was and how perfect the parts were played by the bullies of this lifetime. It was presented that as he forgave the bullies of this lifetime, he was essentially forgiving and freeing himself from lifetimes of guilt. We then thanked all the bullies, the handicap, and the accident for creating this great healing opportunity.

When the session ended, he shared that an enormous feeling of freedom, health and happiness came over him and his back discomfort was "about a zero or one." He was also astonished that he followed the idea of past lives because prior to the session he did not believe in past lives. I asked him why he followed, and he said that it somehow made logical sense at the time and it felt right. A few weeks after the session he reported to his employer that he was ready to return to work.

Leveraging the Utilization of Hypnosis

Because Guided Empathy Meridian Tapping creates new perceptions and neuronal paths regarding old beliefs about certain problematic issues, hypnosis can anchor those new perceptions and the subconscious will interpret them as intention, providing the physiological conditions required for healing. Perception is all we have, and perceptions are accepted by the brain as reality. That "reality" is interpreted by the body and subconscious mind as intention. Our studies have shown that clients who have experienced a shift in a GEMT session will generally be very open to a relaxing guided meditation anchoring what has just transpired.

From the book *My Method* by Emile Coue (1857–1926) is this excerpt: "Even more definite is the doctrine of Aristotle, which taught that 'a vivid imagination compels the body to obey it, for it is a natural principle of movement.'" Coue is called the Father of Applied Conditioning (hypnosis), and he also said, "You have in yourself the instrument of your cure." Contrary to the belief of many, hypnosis was not discovered as a form of entertainment in the old B movies of the 1940s. Avicenna (Ibn Sina) (980–1037), a Persian psychologist and physician, was the earliest to make a distinction between sleep and what is currently known as hypnosis. In *The Book of Healing*, (published in 1027 and recently re-issued as *Avicenna's Medicine, A New Translation*), he referred to hypnosis in Arabic as *al-Wahm al-Amil*, stating that one could create conditions in another person so that he/she accepts the reality (the suggestions) of hypnosis. Better research methods and technologies in recent years have brought mind/body medicine and hypnosis more into the public eye, and they are now accepted as neuroscience.

Anchoring Positive Suggestions

When a client accepts a new, healthier and vastly different perspective about her traumatic childhood event, she will often experience a mild state of hypnosis or trance for a brief time. When this shift occurs, it presents an opportunity to create an anchor for the client so she can continue her positive shift after the session. An anchor can be a physical action associated with a thought and/or feeling while in a hypnotic state for the purpose of recalling it when in a conscious and alert state (post-hypnotic suggestion). For example, "Any time I tap my collarbone I experience that good feeling of forgiveness, knowing that I am also forgiving myself."

Anchoring Self-Responsibility for Future Experiences

When the client understands that she will have to either forgive or find the value in potential future difficult situations, she will do what she can to avoid them. This proactive approach indicates self-responsibility which can greatly improve the quality of life for the client. Prior to the end of the GEMT session, you can empathetically guide the client to the idea of this proactive approach. Once the GEMT portion of the session is complete, hypnosis can be used to anchor this perspective.

Final Step of a GEMT Session

Following a completed session of GEMT and after the final SUDS has been established, you can create a post-hypnotic suggestion to anchor the results of the session. Whether you are a professional certified hypnotherapist, or any other health care practitioner or healer, you can use the following example to apply a hypnotherapy induction following a GEMT session:

Conversing with the client, reflecting on a positive emotion she identified during the GEMT session, ask what color that emotion might be inside her body. (e.g., love and pink)

1. Ask the client to sit back, close her eyes and begin to relax.
2. Suggest that the client remember (or make believe she is in) the deepest trance or relaxation she has ever experienced and ask her to nod her head when she is there or as close to it as possible right now. (This is a form of rapid induction) Wait until you see her nod. (It may take seconds or, rarely, up to a minute.)
3. Apply this or some other induction:
   a. *"Because you are deeply relaxed and are experiencing gratitude and new understanding of (original issue/details) your subconscious mind accepts these new truths (name them) and understands them as your intention. You identified toxic emotions associated with your earlier beliefs and chose to change them to the healthy emotions of (e.g., love, gratitude,*

empathy, etc.) and I invite you now to become aware of the beautiful color (mention and describe the color from Step 1, e.g., pink) that now fills your body, now and for all of the 'nows' for the rest of your life. Experience that emotion of (e.g., love) and that beautiful color (e.g., pink) that is (e.g., love) …….. Experience it …. deeply. Place the palm of your hand on your heart as you experience (e.g., love) and its color (e.g., pink) an anchor} …. Experience it deeply…. And from this moment on {post-hypnotic suggestion}, whenever you place your hand on your heart, with the intention for (e.g., love), you now experience the extraordinary feeling of (e.g., love) and (e.g., pink) and your subconscious mind accepts and actualizes this truth, this intention—physically, mentally and emotionally (and spiritually, if appropriate for this client.) This is your true self. I invite you to think this thought, "This is my true self." Think that thought once again…. and in a moment, as I count from 1 to 5, you will come back to full alertness, filled with (e.g., pink love), your true self, easily and effortlessly, 1…2…3…4 taking a deep breath and beginning to open your eyes even more, and 5, fully alert, fully conscious, very good." (Allow time for the client to be alert.)

4. Ask for SUDS again.

Note: The anchor used in the above induction, "placing the hand on the heart", can also be "tapping the collar bone" or "tapping the chin." The idea is to utilize one of the meridian points already stimulated frequently during the GEMT session.

Quiz - Part 4

1) You have identified the ailment, established SUDS and are about to start the session, but the client feels like she has not talked enough about her issue or you have not asked enough questions. What is the best way to handle this situation?
    a) Record the basic details on a notepad and present a summary of main points back to her so she knows she has been heard.
    b) Delicately communicate your intuitive sense of knowing what the real issue is.
    c) Delay starting the session until the client feels she has given you enough information.
    d) Explain that it is best to begin tapping while continuing the conversation and see where things go.

2) The client has repeated the starting point details in empathetic bond. However, as you start to lead with assumptions the client stops repeating. What should you do first?
    a) Pause and check in with the client to see if she is ok.
    b) Stall
    c) Offer contrasting thoughts.
    d) Try a different assumption down a different path.

3) While leading your client you make an erroneous assumption about her ailment and she corrects you. What is the best course of action?
    a) Apologize for the error and try to be more accurate in your assumptions.
    b) Repeat the client's correction verbatim using "I" statements and continue to lead.
    c) Listen empathetically and do not distract her by repeating her own correction back to her.
    d) Pause and summarize the session thus far.

4) You have identified the emotion associated with the current ailment but then you become stuck, not knowing where to go next. What is ideal?
    a) Remind yourself that overreactions are learned before reasoning skills develop in childhood.
    b) Tell the client you are stuck and ask her to lead.
    c) Attempt to extract more details about the current ailment.
    d) Pause the session and check in with the client.

5) Just minutes after starting the session the client is surprised and overwhelmed as she begins remembering a childhood traumatic event she has not thought about in decades. What is the best course of action?
    a) Tell the client "You are going to be alright."
    b) Pause the session and check in with the client.
    c) Make bold intuitive assumptions about the event.
    d) Stall for more processing time and emotional anesthesia.

6) Your client has just fully confronted her childhood core issue while you empathetically validated her feelings, then offered pros and uncertainty. What is the most important statement to make while in an empathetic bond at this time?
    a) "I forgive that person or persons for what they did."
    b) "It was not my or anyone's fault."
    c) "Why would I put myself through this?"
    d) "I take blame for everything that has happened."

7) In empathetic bond, you are intuitively guided to suggest that the enormous value of her childhood traumatic event was to be free of a subconscious guilt that has plagued her for lifetimes. This being the apex of the session, you leverage your empathetic influence and give enormous value to the childhood traumatic event for her to take responsibility for it. What is the ultimate reason for this?

a) To facilitate the client's understanding that she is not a victim.
b) To ultimately fix or remove her original symptoms.
c) So that she can have the ultimate "aha!" moment realizing that we should be thanking those who innocently play healing roles instead of condemning them.
d) To give her ultimate proof that nothing would exist unless it had value.

PART 5 – Fundamental GEMT Elements

"As soon as you start to tell yourself in your perception that you can't do something anymore, then your biological system will adjust to prove you right." — Bruce Lipton

Mind/Body Connection

Heart Coherence

Heart coherence is a measurable state of emotional and energetic alignment when the focus is on positive thought. The numerous benefits include increased ability to manage and recover from stressful situations, improved memory, and greater ability to focus and process information. The heart's magnetic field is more than 100 times stronger than that of the brain and has neurons which send more information to the brain than it receives from the brain. Though breathwork can be helpful, studies show that during the experience of positive emotions, a sine wave-like heart rate pattern oscillating at a frequency around 0.1 Hz naturally emerges without any conscious changes in breathing. In GEMT, we activate heart coherence at the beginning of a session to experience all the aforementioned benefits.

Mirror Neurons

Mirror neurons are a class of neurons that respond to actions observed in others in the same way as if we performed the action ourselves. It is these neurons that hardwire us for empathy. In GEMT, we empathetically offer a plausible beneficial scenario as to why a traumatic event might be chosen. In doing so, the client's mirror neurons fire, providing the client the experience of choosing it.

Stress Response

During a fight-or-flight response, there is a sudden release of hormones which sets off a chain of reactions that increase heart rate, blood pressure, and breathing rate, which can result in dilated pupils, pale or flushed skin and trembling. Experiencing a fight-or-flight response when there is no threat of physical danger is referred to as a stress response. Under these, and chronic stress conditions, the properties of the stress resilience mediator, neuropeptide Y (NPY), are impeded or become out of balance. This inhibits protection against manifesting diseases and coping with stress.

Pain and suffering are products of the mind/body connection in response to stress. The pain we experience is from the feedback loop between the subconscious mind and body consciousness, which may or may not have anything to do with a physical injury. In GEMT, we use bilateral meridian tapping to temporarily desensitize this feedback while offering a cognitive shift in perception.

New Thought

The New Thought movement is based on the teachings and healing methods of Phineas Quimby (1802–1866), who developed a belief system that illness originated in the mind as a result of misbeliefs and that a mind open to infinite intelligence could overcome any illness. New Thought is the cornerstone of countless alternative healing modalities and self-improvement methods and continues to evolve.

Some of the core concepts of New Thought are
- There is one omnipresent infinite Creator.
- Thoughts and beliefs attract their own fulfillment and dictate reality.
- Divinity dwells within each person.
- Unconditional love and healing toward one another are the highest spiritual principles.

We tend to defend our beliefs but not the truth we share that is inside each of us. When we reduce defensiveness and remind clients of the truth, they transcend their beliefs and heal themselves. GEMT stands on the shoulders of New Thought philosophies and modalities, reaching even higher to empower clients to heal themselves while further minimizing the interference of their free will.

Hermetic Principles

Many of us have experienced an extreme reaction like sadness or anger to a point of absurdity, which caused us to laugh at the absurdity of our reaction. This emotional release of sadness or anger swinging to the same level of laughter is like a pendulum. GEMT leverages the pendulum idea by releasing the highest level of victimhood to reach the highest level of self-responsibility. This is a concept known as the Hermetic Principle of Rhythm; the pendulum swing to the right is the measure of the swing to the left. The Hermetic Principles refer to the teachings of "The Kybalion" passed down by Hermes Trismegistus in ancient Egypt. According to these teachings, there are seven laws by which the universe conducts business: Mentalism, Correspondence, Vibration, Polarity, Rhythm, Cause and Effect, and Gender. Six of these laws can be helpful in explaining the fundamental elements of how and why the GEMT method of healing works.

- Mentalism: The All is mind; the universe is mental.
  - Dis-ease and healing are of the mind.
- Correspondence: As above so below: as below, so above.
  - Mental or spiritual healing can heal physically.
- Vibration: Nothing rests; everything moves, vibrates and circles.
  - When vibration changes, perspective on issues changes.
- Polarity: Everything has its pair of opposites.
  - There is an upside for all the past painful events.
- Rhythm: The pendulum swing to the right is the measure of the swing to the left.
  - Releasing the pendulum at the highest level of victimhood produces the highest level of self-responsibility.
- Cause and Effect: Every cause has its effect; every effect has its cause.
  - The dis-ease is the effect; misperception is the cause.

Meridian Tapping as an Anesthesia

Hospitals in China have been using acupuncture as anesthesia for operations since the late 1950s. Research using functional magnetic resonance imaging (fMRI) and positron emission tomography (PT scan) has suggested certain traditional acupuncture points may be linked to the activation of specific centers in the brain and may present an explanation for their association with specific medical conditions in Traditional Chinese Medicine. Studies have shown that acupressure reduces post-surgical nausea and is as effective as topical anesthesia cream in alleviating anticipatory pain, such as withdrawing a blood sample. Since the 1970s, studies show that stimulating the body's meridians can also be used as an anesthesia for anxiety. In all cases, the mind-body desensitization from meridian tapping is temporary. There can be no permanent healing without a cognitive shift reversing classical conditioning.

Desensitization Eases Classical Conditioning Reversal

Much of the pain we experience from fears and phobias are learned reactions through a process called Identification Association Response or classical conditioning. Ivan Pavlov's research on his dog salivating at the sound of a bell provides us with a basic understanding of how fears and phobias are stored in the unconscious mind as reflexes. When something or someone has hurt us once, we tend to avoid that thing or person because we now expect or anticipate suffering. Because a painful reflex is associated as a negative emotion, we say that "negative emotions are stored as disruptions in the body's energy system."

The learned pain response often grows much worse than the original event that caused it because we now have anticipation, and consequently experience "anticipatory" suffering. Many experience this pain as too uncomfortable to learn a new response. However, when the client is exposed to the stimulus while the unconscious reflex is desensitized (with meridian tapping, for example), a new reaction can be learned quickly with much less discomfort. This is the basis of all desensitization therapies.

112

Dorthy's client Ms. C

While teaching a class on GEMT, I asked if anyone would be interested in being a volunteer for my demonstration of the process and a woman, a friend/guest of a student, raised her hand very quickly, with a "Me, me!" verbal reply. The entire class, including her, laughed at her swift response while she explained how desperate she was to be free from a fear that had plagued her for years.

With my invitation, she joined me in front of the class and told this story. "I'm not sure when all of this began but for many years, I have been deathly afraid of frogs. So much so that I will not travel to a new place until I have called the hotel to make sure there are no frogs around or near the hotel. This fear has prevented me from traveling to certain places, oftentimes making my husband very unhappy and making me realize other people have no understanding about phobias. I can't tell you how many tears I have shed over this problem. I feel guilt, anger, shame, and resentment but I can't get rid of it or past it. A neighbor across the street has a stone frog in his front yard, and I cannot walk on that side of the street near his house. I know this sounds silly, but I have no control over it. I even went to a desensitization clinic in Marin last year that cost me $7,000. I left the $7,000 there but not the phobia! My friend Jan invited me to come to this class with her because she thought you might be able to help me."

I assured her that she had the ability to free herself from an old emotion developed at an earlier age which had now manifested as an irrational fear. I explained and shared information about the subconscious mind, how GEMT works, and how her perception of being a victim contributes to her dis-ease called fear. Before I began leading her in Guided Empathy Meridian Tapping points, I asked her to identify the intensity of her fear on a SUDS scale (0-10) and she said it was 20!

After a few minutes of tapping, while focusing on the value of the fear and using GEMT empathetic conversation, she told me the intensity level seemed to be more like a 5, and we continued exploring the value of the fear in relationship to a possible past life again with relevant statements and results including self-responsibility, forgiveness and gratitude. When asked again she reported the intensity level as a 0 on the scale and the surprised and delighted look on her face told the class and me that something wonderful had happened. Her tearful and happy response was, "I can't believe I spent $7000 and a week of my life on something that didn't work and in 15 minutes with you I am free."

A few days later she called to tell me she visited a pet store the day after our session, went into the amphibian section where she put her nose against the glass of the frog habitat, watched them jump around inches from her face and felt no anxiety or fear. This was someone who couldn't walk past a stone frog. The transformation this woman experienced was already within her. Using GEMT's resultant emotional anesthesia allowed her to find the undiscovered value of a fear and the conscious and subconscious understanding that she no longer had a need for it and was never a victim.

The Four Components of the Mind

Sigmund Freud (1856–1939) posited a model of the mind that has stood the test of time: 10% conscious and 90% subconscious and unconscious, though now considered by many scientists at approximately 5% and 95%. In the book *Hypnosis and Hypnotherapy,* published in 2001, Cal Banyan refers to the Critical Factor" as a function of the mind where new information is compared with existing beliefs held in the subconscious mind and is rejected if significantly different. Bypassing the critical factor is one of the main uses of hypnosis and GEMT.

Each area of the mind has its own function.

- **Conscious mind** – thinks
  It rationally utilizes thoughts, memories, feelings, and wishes of which we are aware at any given moment through mental processing and language.

- **Critical Factor** – questions
  The connecting component between the conscious and subconscious mind, it compares the information perceived through our senses to the information stored in the subconscious and is why the subconscious resists change. It protects against changes to the subconscious and starts developing very early in life.

- **Subconscious mind** – tells or directs
  Contains habits, behaviors and beliefs learned from childhood experiences which, once formed, resist change (i.e., maintain "homeostasis"), with an unlimited learning capacity. It controls 90-95% of the mind and motivates to fulfill perceived needs.

- **Unconscious mind** (primitive mind/body consciousness) – reacts
  A reservoir of feelings, urges, memories, and reflexes outside of conscious awareness. The unconscious holds contents that are unacceptable or unpleasant, such as pain, anxiety, or conflict.

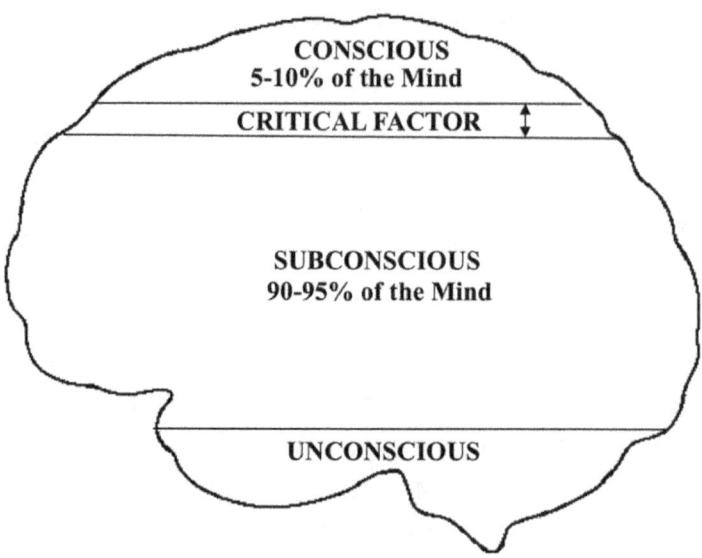

CONSCIOUS
5-10% of the Mind

CRITICAL FACTOR

SUBCONSCIOUS
90-95% of the Mind

UNCONSCIOUS

Difficult situations are often too painful to address. Bilaterally tapping the meridians creates an emotional anesthesia to stop the painful "feedback" from the unconscious to the subconscious. This reduces the pain enough so that the client's subconscious can learn a new perspective from a conscious conversation with a GEMT practitioner. Tapping and bilateral stimulation also relaxes the Critical Factor, allowing changes in the subconscious. The problematic perceptions stored in the subconscious must be found and focused on so they can be neutralized with a new perception. The practitioner uses GEMT techniques, like a detective, to locate the source of these painful emotions, neutralize them, and create a new perspective.

Accessing the Subconscious (Hypnosis or Meridian Tapping)

Two Ways to Access the Subconscious Mind

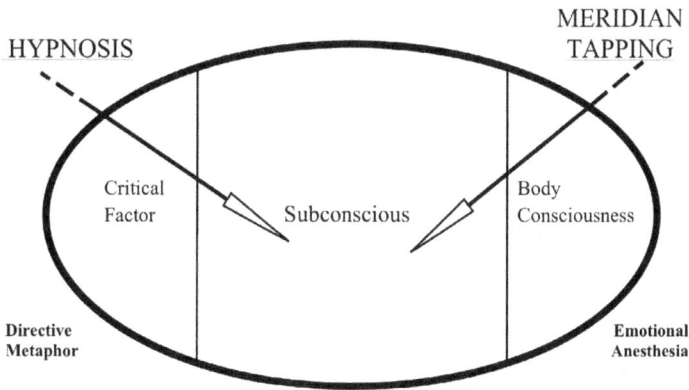

Subconscious Veto (90% of Mind)

The homeostasis principles of the subconscious mind resist changing habits or behaviors because the subconscious associates them with who we are. What we call the "Subconscious Veto" is the dilemma you encounter when consciously wanting to change an aspect that your subconscious perceives as an essential part of you. This includes habits, beliefs, manifestations and, most notably, the identification with victimhood.

The subconscious veto is a fascinating element of this work. For example, many believe that cigarette addiction is from nicotine, or even oral fixation, yet the real struggle around quitting is to no longer identify with it. Cigarette companies fully understand this, as their marketing shows. For example, an ad might display a beautiful day on the lake with friends, with one lovely woman casually holding a cigarette that we can barely see. The cigarette seems to be very much a part of who she is. The smoker and the cigarette are mutually identified. Simply telling a client who wants to quit to hold the cigarette only when taking a drag usually causes considerable resistance. The subconscious sees the act of smoking as a part of who they are, and as a result, will resist dissociating with smoking.

The subconscious, which controls 90% of our mind, often vetoes our conscious decisions by a 9 to 1 ratio. When we see ourselves as victims in life, it is perceived by our subconscious as part of our identity. The healing process of overturning the misperception of victimhood is hindered by the resistance of a subconscious veto. It is also why some people just cannot change, heal, overcome a chronic condition, lose weight, quit smoking, etc., and why they continue to sabotage themselves. We are often unaware that we essentially veto what we consciously want to have happen. Even the most positive person can have the subconscious veto, caused by negative and self-defeating beliefs within the subconscious mind, and it can completely stop any progress. Conscious thinking produces a response and beliefs produce a reaction.

PART 6 – Alternative GEMT Sessions

"You are the eternal creator, never the victim..." —Dr. James Martin
Peebles

Impromptu GEMT Sessions

GEMT sessions can happen almost anywhere at any time. For example, a co-worker/client might experience an acute discomfort while performing day-to-day activities, such as getting an upset stomach from eating a hotdog at a company gathering. In this scenario, an impromptu GEMT session would be appropriate because you might only have a few minutes in an empty conference room to work with your co-worker.

Step-by-Step process of an Impromptu GEMT session

1. Start by suggesting to the client that some acupressure will help ease the discomfort.
2. Find a place nearby that will be free of distractions for 10 minutes
3. Guide the client through the tapping points
4. Suggest that repeating each other while tapping will also help ease the discomfort.
5. State a simple empathetic phrase such as "Well, anyone would have an upset stomach eating that hotdog when stressed."
6. Then, focus on the value without intruding e.g., "The value of this discomfort is to remind me of something, and I don't need to say what that is."
7. Thank the ailment e.g., "I want to thank this upset stomach for the reminder."

That is all that needs to be achieved in an impromptu session. Impromptu sessions typically last less than10 minutes. In our experience, Impromptu sessions have been extremely effective as a remedy for acute discomfort.

Bob's client Ms. A

A client suffering from vitiligo (skin pigmentation disorder) scheduled a GEMT session though she had little expectation that it could help her, especially because the session needed to be done via video conference. Prior to starting the session, she reported her level of discomfort for having the disease for the past few decades was about an 8. We started the session by focusing on the idea that the disease is the perfect metaphor for some past event that was ready to be reframed. The emotions associated with the discomfort of having the vitiligo were shame and guilt. She also felt she was born with the emotions in her skin, which brought up the idea of past lives. She then regressed to when she believed she was a slave, and she believed she was a slave in many previous lives. She felt guilty that she did not free herself when she could in her previous lives, then saw that reflected over and over in her current life. We visualized the shackles unlocked and open, but not leaving the comfort of them. We empathetically healed the guilt using the idea that most humans do this. We then focused on a natural self-love and self-worth that is inside each of us based on a love for freedom and self-responsibility. We brought the idea that she was putting herself in these situations over and over to finally learn the lesson of freedom, a lesson more than worth the discomfort of slavery. We then thanked all the people who, she thought, enslaved her because they were actually helping her learn the value of freedom. After the session the discomfort on the vitiligo was a zero. A few weeks after the session she was ecstatic to share that her vitiligo was about half of what it was prior to the GEMT session. She also reported "the GEMT session helped me heal other parts of myself and life … loving my skin and myself was powerful and helped me make healthier choices to support living a healthier life and my skin's re-pigmentation."

Self-GEMT

Client-practitioner GEMT session is recommended over Self-GEMT, even when the practitioner is unskilled. An empathetic healing journey based in curiosity as to why the practitioner might find her ailment valuable opens and transcends levels of the subconscious. It is far easier to have someone pull us out of a ditch than for us to navigate climbing its walls. However, Self-GEMT can be beneficial when a practitioner is not available, and it does have benefits when desensitizing to the emotion of shame.

Taking the approach of self-responsibility, we can reexamine difficult situations in our lives and see their value, in comparison to not having had them at all. In doing so, we not only realize they have value, but we also discover these events were more than worth the discomfort. We know the value of physical pain is to bring about awareness to stop further damage to the body, like carelessly touching a hot stove. Though we may perceive ourselves as a victim when accidently touching a hot stove, we do not perceive ourselves as a victim of the pain that alerted us to move our hand to prevent further injury. In Self-GEMT we want to bring the ailment created by the subconscious into the foreground of the conscious by treating it as if it were an alert, as in touching a hot stove. The remedy is a result of a negotiation with the subconscious which has been in resistance to parting with the ailment. Metaphorically we ask ourselves, "What hot stove? How am I touching it, and why? What do I need to do?" revealing a specific loving action (forgiveness, acceptance, assistance, kind action, lifestyle adjustment, etc.) to take. The healing shift occurs after the session, when the specified loving action is consciously taken.

Self-GEMT requires a high level of self-honesty. Our questions and statements can be quiet and internal or spoken aloud. Not only do we free ourselves of distractions and raise our vibration, but we also quiet our mind to a meditative state. We give the ailment more than one name/label, if possible, to help reveal its value. Sitting in front of a mirror or self-video conferencing will help maintain the focus on the session.

The healing shift from Self-GEMT occurs after the session; the session itself is not meant to produce a healing shift. Personal love-based answers to the questions and statements during the session become instructions to perform after the session, e.g., modifications in diet, living area, relationship, etc. The willingness and effort to perform the tasks and adjustments will trigger the subconscious healing of the ailment.

Step-by-Step Self-GEMT process

1. Be free of distractions and enter a meditative state.
2. Raise your vibration with a mantra, e.g., "I am the presence of Divine Love."
3. Complete three rounds of tapping to calm any defensiveness.
4. "So, I have this ___." (Give the ailment a few names if possible.)
5. "Nothing would exist unless it had value and this ___ is no exception."
6. "Why am I having this ___ when others are not?"
7. "What qualities do I like about the people who don't have ___?"
8. "There must be a reason why this ___ is more than worth the discomfort."
9. "What emotions are present in this ___?"
10. "When did I first notice having this ___?"
11. "What is the value of having this ___? How is it protecting me?"
12. "Why do I think this ___ is still needed? Where am I still in resistance?"
13. "What do I need to do to resolve this ___?"

From our experience, taking responsibility to perform the specified action revealed from the question "what do I need to do?" will create a healing shift in the subconscious in a way similar to walking a labyrinth. This is a way of asking the subconscious or higher self for the lesson that needs to be learned and the specific action that will prove it was learned. With the willingness to take the specified action, by virtue of intent, a healing shift occurs.

Some example honest answers from the subconscious might be:
- Have lunch with my estranged father/mother.
- Make more self-time to reduce stress or meditate.
- Change posture or diet.
- Clean or organize your office, garage, storage, etc.

The actions to take need to be quantifiable. Subjective actions such as "Stop judging and condemning" or "Show more unconditional love" are not quantifiable. The reasons or actions will not become apparent if the discomfort or disease is devalued. Where you have played the devil's advocate in devaluing the dis-ease, you are now the angel's advocate through compassionate self-reexamination in finding the value. This practice will strengthen your abilities as a GEMT practitioner, your acceptance of self-responsibility, and your belief that you are always the creator of your life experiences.

GEMT by Proxy

Proxy GEMT is empathetically substituting for someone else. It is based on Carl Jung's theory of the Collective Unconscious, and the concept that we are all energetically connected and fundamentally one in Spirit. When someone cannot participate in GEMT themselves, you or someone else can assume the role for that person by proxy. The only requirement to act as a proxy is that you recognize and feel a connection to the one for whom you are substituting. You become the client, in a manner of speaking. Proxy GEMT works for anyone: babies, small children, people with dementia, the physically weak, those who are handicapped, and those too ill to tap for themselves. It can also work for pets or plants, because proxy GEMT can be equated to the intention of prayer.

The proxy simply sets the intention through spoken words or thought. Start by designating the session to one intended to receive the benefits i.e., "This session is for _____." The proxy empathetically "puts herself in the place of the child, person, animal, or plant." This means responding, as best they can, with words that the child, person, animal, or plant might say if they could express their feelings in words. It is important to "tune-in" to the emotions or state of distress of the other being that the session is intending to relieve.

It's important for the proxy to "stay out of the way." The proxy's attention and intention should be free of personal views, opinions and expectations. Keeping a clear and receptive mind is required to be a good proxy. It may be helpful to have direct physical contact (touching hands) between the proxy and the person being served. This can make the connection very clear to the proxy's mind.

The intensity level of the problem can be gauged by observing the client. Observe the behavior, mood, rigidity of the body, voice tone, tenseness in posture, energy level, facial expressions, and other gestures. Be aware of any changes to determine if the intensity is decreasing or losing its charge. Sighing, yawning, rapid blinking, burping, and even flatulence are all good signs of "energy release."

Proxy GEMT Over the Phone or with Video Conference

The idea is the same, though over the phone the practitioner would need to call out the current tapping point when it changes. For example, a person calls and is unable to speak or listen clearly because she is overwhelmed with emotional upset. You as the practitioner would set the intention: "This proxy session is for _____ (the person on the line)." Throughout the session, empathetically and intuitively communicate her actions and feelings, e.g., "tapping on my eyebrow," "I am feeling stressed" while focusing on her as if she were sitting across from you. Once she is calm enough to give you information, regular GEMT can be used.

Proxy GEMT Over the Phone or Video with the Caller as the Proxy

The child, a person with dementia, or a person too physically ill to talk or move may be with the caller. It is helpful if the caller can be next to or touching the person being served. Because the caller is most likely the person asking for help on behalf of the client, it is important to "tune in" to the caller as they "tune in" to the client. The proxy will need to be your eyes and ears and give you feedback on intensity and any noticeable changes. You may need to ask several questions of the proxy. In this case, it may be helpful to know how to do self-muscle testing using yourself as the proxy (Dr. George Goodheart, Applied Kinesiology). More accurate information can be gained when you are well practiced and trained in this art.

124

EPILOGUE

"It is reasonable to expect the doctor to recognize that science may not have all the answers to problems of health and healing." —Norman Cousins

If you follow the steps for Guided Empathy Meridian Tapping and understand the philosophical theories comprising its foundation, we are confident that you will "make a difference," not only in the lives of yourself and others, but in the world. Practice is the main component in any new procedure to make it your own, and that is our objective; how you do this becomes your own personal approach to GEMT. We don't know your story and why you decided to read this book or take this course, but we do know your life contained transformational moments in your journey to become a healer. As you reflect on those moments in your life, you know when you changed from who you were to who you were becoming, and it is those transformational moments that connect us all as healers.

The Great Cosmic Web of Choices – Bob's Personal Story

It was a beautiful afternoon, and I was walking home from junior high school through its big open field. When I got to the center of the field, a huge wave of unconditional love hit me, somehow letting me know I am exactly where I should be in every aspect of my life and that everything is somehow perfect.

I somehow knew that where I am physically as well as all the situations of my life are the product of my choices, which are choices made in response to other choices, which are choices based on other choices, going back to the beginning of time. For example, the road could have been made where I am standing now, and the center of the field could be where the road is now. Everything is a choice whether deliberate or unconscious, based on a previous choice, whether deliberate or unconscious. If anything was different than it is now, even the way a blade of grass is growing, things would not be exactly the way they are now. Yet this is the perfect exact state.

All choices are based on other choices and are the framework of future choices. All of life is bound together by the great cosmic web of reactive choices. I felt the truth that all past choices are perfectly unchangeable, for it is the foundation of this perfect moment. I realized that if I ever attack or regret past choices, then I am not seeing this moment as perfect. When I do accept the past, I know I am exactly where I should be.

Lessons Learned, Life to Live – Dorthy's Personal Story

Years ago, when I lived and worked in Syracuse, N.Y., my best friend from high school and college called me to tell me she and her family were moving back to California, and she wanted me to move there with them. This call came about two weeks after I had looked up to the Heavens and pleadingly shouted, "Get me out of here!" That plea came from me because I was in a difficult relationship and, at that time in my life, didn't have the consciousness, courage or strength to end it. Only in retrospect did I see the correlation between my plea and the phone call because at that time I only experienced an overpowering fear, which surprised me, as my reaction to the call. I told her I would have to think about it and call her back in two weeks. Needless to say, I looked for every reason I could conjure to convince myself of the necessity to stay in Syracuse with everything "I knew." I asked everyone and anyone for advice, I looked for excuses and reasons to not go, I deliberated, I rationalized, I exhausted myself.

After all the advice and suggestions, the rationalizations and deliberations, I finally admitted to myself my fear was the problem. I had no reason not to go to California, or anyplace else for that matter! I was "as free as the breeze" as the saying goes. The evening before I was to call my friend back, I was sitting in my living room thinking about what I was going to say, what excuse I would give about not going, without admitting to the fear, when I felt a sense of calm deep inside me. I had felt that calm only once before during a very spiritual and personal moment in my life.

As I sat back on the sofa and closed my eyes, I heard these words: "When you don't do something because you're afraid to, you will never be the same again." The words were like a thought I was hearing, but not my thought; it was a man's voice. Guardian angel? Spirit guide? Divine Intelligence? In retrospect I would say Guide, but who can know for sure?

The one thing I do know for sure is that those words changed my life forever. I called my friend, and rather than making excuses, I said "Yes", and within a few weeks I was on my way to California and all the experiences, opportunities, joys, lessons, and personal evolutions that only saying "Yes" can provide.

Self-forgiveness - The Healing Journey

As I continue to raise my consciousness,
I increasingly become aware of my unconscious actions and behaviors,
all of which I must forgive.
If I resist forgiving myself,
I attract those behaviors and actions upon me, time and time again.
These experiences can generate *retaliation*, *anger* and *resentment*
but these emotions have a higher vibration than that of *guilt*.
I have chosen these experiences to provide a catalyst for self-forgiveness.
I forgive myself as I forgive another.
I can recall moments when I felt no need to retaliate
when I was attacked.
This indicates I have no guilt about those specific actions and behaviors.
It is essential, though, that I recognize my grievances
and feelings of vengeance as a beacon,
alerting and guiding me on my journey to my long-awaited self-
forgiveness.
When I view my negative emotions as a gold mine
for healing my own guilt,
I can then thank my attacker for playing his role,
and simply say,
"I forgive myself for every time I have done something similar"
My *peace* and *invulnerability* are restored in this greater awareness of
I am that *I Am*.

Thank you,

Robert Ranche and Dorthy Tyo

"This game can only be won by those who lose their cards in the melting influence of love; can only be won by those who lay their pleasures, their limitations, their all upon the table face up and say inwardly: 'All, all of you players, each other-self, whatever your hand, I love you.' This is the game: to know, to accept, to forgive, to balance, and to open the self in love. This cannot be done without the forgetting, for it would carry no weight in the life of the mind/body/spirit beingness totality." – The Law of One

Appendix

GEMT Session Transcripts

Sample GEMT Session - A (From 8 to 0 SUDs Back Pain in 15 Minutes)

This is a transcript of an actual GEMT session and a good example of how a session can go (P is Practitioner, C is Client).

Step 1 – Raise client's vibration/mood.
1. P: Okay (client's name), close your eyes and take a nice deep breath. Think about all the people you love and that love you. Raise your vibration as high as possible, aligning yourself with your higher self. Feeling that run through your body and it feels good, in complete alignment. And as you're feeling that high vibration, gently open your eyes when you're ready.

Step 2 – Get starting point issue (What, When, SUDS).
2. P: What would you like to work on today?
3. C: Can we work on pain?
4. P: Pain?
5. C: More emotional.
6. P: Okay.
7. C: Well, I have this pain right here on my back on the side and I know it has something to do with some emotion because it keeps getting displaced.
8. P: Mmm. On a 0 to 10 scale where would you put the intensity?
9. C: About 7 or 8. It goes from my knee to my back and just moves around so I know it has something to do with some emotion, but I can't figure it out.
10. P: Ok, and how long has it been in your back location?
11. C: Six months now.
12. P: Okay, and prior to that it was in the knee, okay. And how long was it there?
13. C: A couple of years.
14. P: Mmmm. A couple of years.

15. C: Or more.
16. P: And prior to that?
17. C: I don't remember where it was.
18. P: And so, this is back three years ago, four years ago?
19. C: I see that when my son was born, I started having this pain. Right around that time. My son is 10 now and it started slowly, and it became worse over time. And, about six months ago I started working on this and it would just move from here (knee) to my back.

Step 3 – Start tapping and explaining GEMT and tapping.

20. P: Mmm. That's fantastic. (Tapping starts.) Let's start with it here (tapping on side of palm). So, we tap on the meridian points of the body to balance the body's energy system. So, this is the first one, the side of your palm. And then to the top of the head. Very, very good. You must have done this before.
21. C: Mmm-hmm.
22. P: Eyebrows. And then the side of the eye. You might be feeling your body begin to balance already. And here (while tapping under eye). So, the only reason we do this is to be able to have a conversation about anything without getting defensive. For example, if I was to tell you that wall was purple and you weren't tapping, you might say 'Hey, you are trying to pull a fast one on me! That wall is yellow!' but now that we're tapping, you're just going to say, 'No it's not, it's yellow.' And that's why we tap. So, when I say things, you can correct me and not get defensive. Because I don't know. I'm trying to learn what it's like to be you. So, this will help us speed up the process of me understanding what it's like to have a pain in my knee and then a pain in my back in a very specific area. Repeating after me in I statements, and then you take the lead, when you feel like it, correcting me whenever.

Step 4 – Begin Empathetic Bond.

23. P: Nothing would exist
24. C: Nothing would exist
25. P: Unless it had value.
26. C: Unless it had value.

Step 5 – Say what you know about the issue.

130

27.   P: And right now, this pain in my back
28.   C: And right now, this pain in my back
29.   P: Is no exception.
30.   C: Is no exception.
31.   P: It absolutely has value.
32.   C: It absolutely has value.
33.   P: Prior to that,
34.   C: Prior to that,
35.   P: When it was in my knee,
36.   C: When it was in my knee,
37.   P: It also had value.
38.   C: It also had value.
39.   P: Focusing on where it's right now. As I focus on where it's on right now,
40.   C: As I focus on where it's on right now,
41.   P: As I'm focusing on this pain,
42.   C: As I'm focusing on this pain,

Step 7 – Build client trust and learn about the issue

43.   P: I'm noticing a particular emotional element to it.
44.   C: I'm noticing a particular emotional element to it.
45.   P: Because all physical pain
46.   C: Because all physical pain
47.   P: Has an emotional element to it.
48.   C: Has an emotional element to it.
49.   P: And the pain in my back is no exception.
50.   C: And the pain in my back is no exception.
51.   P: So, this emotional element.
52.   C: So, this emotional element.
53.   P: This emotional aspect.
54.   C: This emotional aspect.
55.   P: Is
56.   C: Is

Step 8 – Define the emotion

57.   P: I want to define it as
58.   C: I want to define it as

59. P: The emotion of
60. C: The emotion of
61. (Pause and wait for client)
62. C: Fear and anxiety.
63. P: Fear and anxiety. I have fear and anxiety in my back.
64. C: I have fear and anxiety in my back.
65. P: And when I say that,
66. C: And when I say that,
67. P: It feels right.
68. C: It feels right.
69. P: I already know I'm exactly where I need to be right now in life.
70. C: I already know I'm exactly where I need to be right now in life.
71. P: Right here right now.
72. C: Right here right now.
73. P: Looking at this issue.
74. C: Looking at this issue.
75. P: Ready to come forward.
76. C: Ready to come forward.
77. P: I know
78. C: I know
79. P: This fear and anxiety
80. C: This fear and anxiety
81. P: Has a familiar aspect to it.
82. C: Has a familiar aspect to it.
83. P: Like listening to a song
84. C: Like listening to a song
85. P: From long ago.
86. C: From long ago.
87. P: As I pay attention to this emotional element
88. C: As I pay attention to this emotional element
89. P: Coming from my back,
90. C: Coming from my back,

Step 9 – Take the client back to the childhood event

91. P: It reminds me of where I had this before,
92. C: It reminds me of where I had this before,

132

93. P: When I was a child.
94. C: When I was a child.
95. P: And, where am I?
96. C: I see my dad.
97. P: I see my dad. And what is my dad doing?
98. C: He's mad.
99. P: He's mad, again?
100. C: Yes.
101. P: He's mad again.
102. C: He's mad again.
103. P: My dad is mad again.
104. C: My dad is mad again.
105. P: Why would he be mad?
106. C: He's just like that.
107. P: He's just like that. Why did he need to be mad, who knows.
108. C: Why did he need to be mad, who knows.
109. P: Why did I sign up for that?
110. C: Why did I sign up for that?
111. P: I didn't do anything wrong.
112. C: I didn't do anything wrong.
113. P: It is unjust.
114. C: It is unjust.
115. P: And even he knew it.
116. C: And even he knew it.
117. P: Anytime I get a little frustrated
118. C: Anytime I get a little frustrated
119. P: With my son,
120. C: With my son,
121. P: I'm reminded
122. C: I'm reminded
123. P: Of how not to be.
124. C: Of how not to be.
125. P: For indeed
126. C: For indeed
127. P: I am NOT my father.

128. C: I am NOT my father.
129. P: I wish I had a father like me.
130. C: I wish I had a father like me.
131. P: I am doing such a good job.
132. C: I am doing such a good job.

Step 10 – Ask "Why would I put myself through this?"

133. P: Yet what about my father?
134. C: Yet what about my father?
135. P: Why did I pick him?
136. C: Why did I pick him?

Step 11 – Offer a valuable reason for choosing the event

137. P: A way to prepare me
138. C: A way to prepare me
139. P: To be
140. C: To be
141. P: The best father now.
142. C: The best father now.
143. P: Such a tough life,
144. C: Such a tough life,
145. P: But it worked.
146. C: But it worked.

Step 12 – Thank the childhood event and the people involved

147. P: I should thank him.
148. C: I should thank him.
149. P: And I do.
150. C: And I do.
151. P: I know for certain
152. C: I know for certain
153. P: That I will never be that way to my son.
154. C: That I will never be that way to my son.

Step 13 – Thank the original issue

155. P: And I want to thank my back,
156. C: And I want to thank my back,
157. P: The pain in my back.
158. C: The pain in my back.

134

159. P: It was the pain in my knee,
160. C: It was the pain in my knee,
161. P: For bringing it to my attention
162. C: For bringing it to my attention
163. P: That I need to free him
164. C: That I need to free him
165. P: And thank him
166. C: And thank him
167. P: For conditioning me
168. C: For conditioning me
169. P: To be what I think
170. C: To be what I think
171. P: Is the perfect father.
172. C: Is the perfect father.
173. P: The school of hard knocks,
174. C: The school of hard knocks,
175. P: I lived it
176. C: I lived it
177. P: In perfection.
178. C: In perfection.
179. P: I'm happy to be here.
180. C: I'm happy to be here.
181. P: I'm exactly where I need to be.
182. C: I'm exactly where I need to be.
183. P: I'm going to help my son
184. C: I'm going to help my son
185. P: To be a perfect father like me.
186. C: To be a perfect father like me.
187. P: Then I turn into the perfect grandpa.
188. C: Then I turn into the perfect grandpa.
189. P: All is well in the world.
190. C: All is well in the world.

Step 14 – Stop tapping and get SUDS

191. (Continue tapping one round, no talking. Then tapping stops) … End of session.

192. P: So, how are you doing?
193. C: Oh my gosh.
194. P: Do you remember the SUDS level of your back pain prior to the session?
195. C: Seven or eight?
196. P: Ok, And now maybe?
197. C: Right now, I don't feel right now. I feel some residue except that I know something was there and it's not there anymore. almost like a hollowness. Like a tube.
198. P: Oh, okay.
199. C: That goes from here (knee) to here (back), all the way up my back.
200. P: That's fantastic!
201. C: I have no idea how you did this, really. It was just, like, bam flash, flash. I noticed that in myself, all of a sudden, that was freedom right there. I got the cage open, I just felt, I just felt free. I have done this in psychotherapy— this, this goes at a different level and so instantaneously. There are no words to explain it. I want to call him (my father) and tell them that I love him. I am conscious and aware of my emotions all the time because I do a lot of work. I never thought that this is going to go this way. I have absolutely no idea where this is going to go, and that's why this is a miracle. I call this a miracle.

Notes on Sample Session - A

In this first sample session, we can see that GEMT is simply a conversation. This client is a healer and is already familiar with the healing process of correcting misperceptions that typically speed up sessions considerably. Rapid sessions such as this one often don't have a "Step 6 - Make assumptions and repeat corrections," or a "Step 15 – Anchor healing with hypnotherapy," though those steps are extremely important in slower sessions. Lines 163–172 revisit the idea of thanking who he was previously condemning, which can be done multiple times in a session.

Sample GEMT Session - B (From 9 to 2 SUDs Undisclosed Sadness in 15 Minutes)

This is a transcript of an actual GEMT session. The session demonstrates that healing can still occur even though a client does not want to reveal details about the childhood source issue (P is Practitioner, C is Client).

Step 1 – Raise client's vibration/mood.
1. P: Okay (client's name), take a nice easy breath in and gently close your eyes and think about all the people that have ever loved you and you love in your life. Bringing all that into the present moment, raising your vibration as high as you possibly can, connecting to your higher source, elevating enough. You are one with all the omni-present energy in every part of your body, every cell, every molecule. When you feel that, gently come back into the room and gently open your eyes.

Step 2 – Get starting point issue (What, When, SUDS).
2. P: What would you like to work on today?
3. C: Sadness
4. P: Sadness, that's excellent. And where would you put that on a scale of 0 to 10?
5. C: Nine
6. P: A nine, that's excellent. and how long have you had this sadness?
7. C: Umm, forever.
8. P: Forever, as far back as you can remember.
9. C: Umm, yeah.
10. P: Ok, that's excellent. and does it come and go. does it …
11. C: Yes.
12. P: It does come and go.
13. C: Now, yes.

Step 3 – Start tapping and explaining GEMT and tapping.
14. P: Very, very good. Okay let's start tapping here.
15. (3 rounds of tapping …)

Step 4 – Begin Empathetic Bond.
16. P: So, I've had this sadness for a while.
17. C: So, I've had this sadness for a while.

Step 5 – Say what you know about the issue.

18. P: It comes and goes.
19. C: It comes and goes.
20. P: I've had it for a while.
21. C: I've had it for a while.
22. P: In fact, as long as I can remember.
23. C: In fact, as long as I can remember.
24. P: Certain times in my life,
25. C: Certain times in my life,
26. P: It comes up again.
27. C: It comes up again.
28. P: Other times I forget about it.
29. C: Other times I forget about it.

Step 6 – Make assumptions and repeat corrections.

30. P: But I know it's always there. or not.
31. C: Oh no.
32. P: I don't always know it's there.
33. C: No, I don't always know it's there.
34. P: Because ...
35. C: Because it's getting better.

Step 7 – Build client trust and learn about the issue.

36. P: Because it's getting better, I've noticed it's getting better.
37. C: I've noticed it's getting better.
38. P: And the reason why it's getting better
39. C: And the reason why it's getting better
40. P: Is ...
41. C: There's a lot of personal work.
42. P: There's a lot of personal work. That helps me look at
43. C: That helps me look at

Step 8 – Define the emotion.

44. P: The sadness.
45. C: The sadness.
46. P: The core issue.
47. C: The core issue.

Step 9 – Take the client back to the childhood event.

48. P: Long ago,
49. C: Long ago,
50. P: For it would have to be,
51. C: It would have to be.
52. P: If I have had this for a long time,
53. C: If I have had this for a long time,
54. P: Then it must have been around since long ago.
55. C: Oh yeah, long ago.
56. P: I must have been a little girl.
57. C: I was.
58. P: I was, I actually remember.
59. C: Yes, I remember.
60. P: I remember where it all started.
61. C: Yes, I remember where it all started.
62. P: Especially a big part of it.
63. C: Especially a big part of it.
64. P: Actually, it happened in one situation.
65. C: Yeah, it happened in one situation.
66. P: Or not maybe it didn't happen in one situation.
67. C: It did happen in one situation.
68. P: It did happen in one situation; I'm remembering more clearly now.
69. C: I'm remembering more clearly now.
70. P: Could be because I feel more comfortable about remembering it. I'm allowing myself
71. C: I'm allowing myself
72. P: To remember it more
73. C: To remember it more
74. P: Because I'm more calm.
75. C: Because I'm more calm.
76. P: And that's okay.
77. C: And that's okay.
78. P: I'm telling myself
79. C: I'm telling myself
80. P: That it's okay.

81.   C: It's okay.
82.   P: I'm following you.
83.   C: And I'm trying.
84.   P: You're doing so good.
85.   C: Yes, but it's big stuff.
86.   P: It's big stuff. I remember the situation.
87.   C: I remember the situation, but I'm not sure I want to talk about it
88.   P: But I'm not sure I want to talk about it.
89.   C: I'm not sure I want to talk about it.
90.   P: I'm not sure I want to talk about it because
91.   C: I'm not sure I want to talk about it because... I feel vulnerable.
92.   P: I feel vulnerable.
93.   C: About it.
94.   P: I feel vulnerable about it. I'm giving myself
95.   C: I'm giving myself
96.   P: Self-respect
97.   C: Self-respect
98.   P: To be okay
99.   C: To be okay
100. P: About not wanting to talk about it.
101. C: About not wanting to talk about it.
102. P: I'm okay with that.
103. C: I'm okay with that.
104. P: I'm okay with not wanting to talk about it.
105. C: I'm okay with not wanting to talk about it.
106. P: I can talk about it in a different way.
107. C: I can talk about it in a different way, yes.
108. P: That might help me.
109. C: That might help me.
110. P: I might make up a name or a sound for it.
111. C: Umm ...
112. P: Or an object
113. C: Umm ....
114. P: Or a color.
115. C: It is something that would feel good?

140

116. P: It is something that would feel good. I can have it be whatever way I want it to be.
117. C: Umm ...
118. P: I'm allowing myself
119. C: I'm allowing myself
120. P: To be myself.
121. C: To be myself.
122. P: To accept myself.
123. C: To accept myself.
124. P: I've done a lot of work with this.
125. C: I've done a lot of work with this.
126. P: I've created all these paths to it.
127. C: I've created all these paths to it.
128. P: And I'm recognizing that now.
129. C: And I'm recognizing that now.
130. P: And what I really want to
131. C: And what I really want to
132. P: Is just be okay with the situation.
133. C: Just be okay with the situation, and I guess, find the value to it.
134. P: And find the value to it, and that will be very good for me.
135. C: And that would be very good for me and my children.
136. P: And my children.
137. C: Um hm.
138. P: As I tap,
139. C: As I tap,
140. P: I tap for them in mind,
141. C: I tap for them in mind,
142. P: Because my healing
143. C: Because my healing
144. P: Can affect them.
145. C: Can affect them, and will heal them.
146. P: And will heal them, because somehow, they are affected by this as well.
147. C: Because they're affected by this as well.
148. P: Even though it happened before they were born.

149. C: Even though it happened before they were born.
150. P: Great healing has already occurred
151. C: Great healing has already occurred
152. P: By me accepting the situation.
153. C: By me accepting the situation.
154. P: Nothing would exist
155. C: Nothing would exist
156. P: Unless it had value.
157. C: Unless it had value.
158. P: And that sad episode long ago
159. C: And that sad episode long ago
160. P: That I'm not going to talk about
161. C: No
162. P: But, that sad episode long ago, is absolutely valuable.
163. C: Because I am here today.
164. P: Because I am here today.
165. C: So happy to be here.
166. P: So happy to be here. I see the value is beyond my comprehension.
167. C: I see the value is beyond my comprehension.
168. P: It has been enormous for my spiritual growth.
169. C: It has been enormous for my spiritual growth.
170. P: Because I know now what's more true
171. C: Because I know now what's more true
172. P: Is that my true strength
173. C: Is that my true strength
174. P: Comes from source energy
175. C: Comes from source energy
176. P: And not from the body
177. C: And not from the body
178. P: Or this planet.
179. C: Or this planet.
180. P: I have the power
181. C: I have the power
182. P: To create mountains.
183. C: To create mountains.

184. P: To create universes,
185. C: To create universes,
186. P: If I would just accept it.
187. C: If I would just accept it.

Step 10 – Ask "Why would I put myself through this?"

188. P: And I created that situation
189. C: And I created that situation

Step 11 – Offer a valuable reason for choosing the event

190. P: To bring to my awareness,
191. C: To bring to my awareness,
192. P: My power,
193. C: My power,
194. P: To heal
195. C: To heal
196. P: Under extreme circumstances.
197. C: Under extreme circumstances.
198. P: And indeed, I am so proud.
199. C: And indeed, I am so proud.
200. P: That is why I am a healer.
201. C: That is why I am a healer.
202. P: Because I want to help others
203. C: Because I want to help others
204. P: Who have gone through what I have gone through.
205. C: Who have gone through what I have gone through.
206. P: For I am the only one
207. C: For I am the only one
208. P: Who can help them.
209. C: Who can help them.
210. P: Many are called,
211. C: Many are called,
212. P: Few answer.
213. C: Few answer.
214. P: And I've been called.
215. C: And I've been called.
216. P: And I answered.

217. C: And I answered.

(again) Step 10 – Ask "Why would I put myself through this?"

218. P: Before I incarnated,
219. C: Before I incarnated,
220. P: I needed to go through this.
221. C: I needed to go through this.

Step 12 – Thank the childhood event and the people involved.

222. P: I so want to thank
223. C: I so want to thank
224. P: Those players from that time long ago.
225. C: My mother.
226. P: My mother, I want to thank my mother.
227. C: I want to thank my mother.
228. P: Because she helped me be
229. C: Because she helped me be
230. P: The great healer I am today.
231. C: The great healer I am today.
232. P: I would not change a thing.
233. C: I would not change a thing.
234. P: I am the creator of my reality.
235. C: I am the creator of my reality.
236. P: I am the creator of all my experiences.
237. C: I am the creator of all my experiences.
238. P: Including the one as a child.
239. C: Including the one as a child.
240. P: For I have grown by leaps and bounds
241. C: For I have grown by leaps and bounds
242. P: This lifetime.
243. C: This lifetime.
244. P: I am a great powerful healer
245. C: I am a great powerful healer
246. P: Thanks to school of hard knocks.
247. C: Thanks to school of hard knocks.
248. P: Thanks to the difficult time I went through as a child.
249. C: Thanks to the difficult time I went through as a child.

Step 13 – Thank the original issue (undisclosed – implied).

250. P: I'll just tap for a little bit. Very very good. I've been true to myself in this session.
251. C: I've been true to myself in this session.
252. P: I feel honored
253. C: I feel honored
254. P: And respected
255. C: And respected
256. P: And I've done well.
257. C: And I've done well.
258. P: Taking a deep breath, relaxing, I am exactly where I should be.
259. C: I am exactly where I should be.
260. (Tapping stops)

Step 14 – Stop tapping and get SUDS.

261. P: How are you?
262. C: I'm good
263. P: On a scale of zero to ten, where would you put that whatever that was, sadness?
264. C: Umm, down, maybe a 2.
265. P: Maybe a 2, that's very, very good. What would you like to share about your experience being a client?
266. C: It's a topic that has been coming back and so it's amazing to get a new approach to it. and it's a little bit more healing because it's, even though a lot of work, and a lot of different ways to work on it, and around it, just a different and different approach and. I don't know. it's all I can say for now. I am sure things will unfold and settle in. Thank you.
267. P: Thank you.

Notes on Sample Session - B

This GEMT session was a classroom demonstration with a student as a client. She did not feel comfortable getting into too much detail in front of her friends and classmates. This session shows that GEMT can be effective with little detail about the ailment or discomfort.

Sample GEMT Session - C (From 8 to 0 SUDS Anxiety in 30 Minutes)

This is a transcript of an actual GEMT session. The session demonstrates that discomfort can move to a related childhood core issue (P is Practitioner, C is Client).

Step 1 – Raise client's vibration/mood.

1. P: Okay (client's name), take a nice, deep, gentle breath in, and gently close your eyes, relaxing into your body, raising your vibration, thinking of all the people you love and that love you in all of your lifetimes for eternity. Bringing all the loving energy of every lifetime into the present moment, feeling that love, feeling that connection to the source energy, raising your vibration as high as you possibly can, feeling it in every cell of your body, and how natural it feels, feeling the loving vibration and gently taking a deep breath in. And when you are ready, gently open your eyes and come back into the room.

Step 2 – Get starting point issue (What, When, SUDS).

2. P: What would you like to work on today?
3. C: I was recently in a car accident and I am having a lot of anxiety related to that.
4. P: Okay, and how long ago was the car accident?
5. C: In March
6. P: Okay and on a scale of zero to ten where would you put this discomfort about this card accident?
7. C: Seven
8. P: A seven, That's very, very good, okay. So, March would be just about two months ago, right?
9. C: March, About a month and a half ago.
10. P: About a month and a half ago, about six weeks ago; prior to that you were fine driving.
11. C: Yes
12. P: That's very, very good, and you put that on the scale at about seven.
13. C: Right.

Step 3 – Start tapping and explaining GEMT and tapping.

146

14. P: Let's start out with tapping points. We tap on the meridian points of the body to balance the body's energy system. That's the first one, side of palm, a second one will be on the top of the head. A lot of people like it. Eyebrows. That's very,very good. Side of the eye, and then underneath the pupil about one inch below the pupil. And the indentation of the chin. We tap on the meridian points of the body, that's the collar bone, on the side here, four to six inches below the armpit. We tap on the meridian points of the body so we can have a conversation about anything and not get too defensive. For example, if I was to say this wall was purple and you weren't tapping, you might get too defensive and wonder why I would start with a statement like that. But if we are tapping you would just say, "No it's not purple, it's white." And that's the kind of conversation we have while we tap. It's a normal conversation without getting defensive. And so, the purpose of our conversation is for me to understand what it's like to be you. To be upset about that car accident. So, you're going to teach me what it's like to experience what you experience and sometimes you'll lead and sometimes I'll lead and when I lead, and I make a mistake, you correct me. No big deal because we're tapping. I'm just trying to learn what it's like. It gives you the opportunity to see your discomfort about the car accident in me.

15. C: I want to say, about the number I gave. It's higher than a seven.
16. P: Oh, it's higher than seven. Okay, how high is it?
17. C: It's at least an eight. I feel it in my body.
18. P: You feel it in your body. and what about in your body?
19. C: In my chest.
20. P: In your chest, that's very, very good. So, you feel the discomfort as an eight in your body. Okay and could it be an emotion that's with that feeling in your chest?
21. C: Like anger.
22. P: Like anger, that's very, very good. So, this is excellent. I'm going to start talking in the "I statements" as if it was me who had this, and you can repeat after me to follow me and then correct me.

Step 4 – Begin Empathetic Bond.

23.   P: So, right now,
24.   C: Right now,
25.   P: I've noticed
26.   C: I've noticed

Step 5 – Say what you know about the issue.

27.   P: That the discomfort from the car accident
28.   C: That the discomfort from the car accident
29.   P: Is in my chest.
30.   C: Is in my chest.
31.   P: And it's about an eight.
32.   C: And it's about an eight.
33.   P: And it's about an eight in anger.
34.   C: And it's about an eight in anger.

Step 6 – Make assumptions and repeat corrections.

35.   P: And it's very particular anger.
36.   C: And it's very particular anger.

Step 7 – Build client trust and learn about the issue.

37.   P: It's very unique.
38.   C: It's very unique.
39.   P: It's very familiar.
40.   C: It's very familiar.
41.   P: It reminds me
42.   C: It reminds me

Step 8 – Define the emotion.

43.   P: That I've had this type of anger before.
44.   C: That I've had this type of anger before.
45.   P: I am angry because of something particular.
46.   C: I am angry because of something particular.
47.   P: I actually know what that is.
48.   C: I actually know what that is.
49.   P: I'm angry because
50.   C: I'm angry because
51.   P: Something's not fair.
52.   C: Something's not fair.
53.   P: Something's not right.

54. C: Something's not right.
55. P: Something's not justified.
56. C: Something's not justified.
57. P: Something's not fair.
58. C: Something's not fair.

Step 9 – Take the client back to the childhood event.

59. P: And like a familiar song from long ago
60. C: And like a familiar song from long ago
61. P: That can transport me back in time,
62. C: That can transport me back in time,
63. P: I remember as a child
64. C: I remember as a child
65. P: When I felt that same anger.
66. C: When I felt that same anger.
67. P: And where am I?
68. C: My sister.
69. P: My sister
70. C: My sister
71. P: Has made me angry
72. C: Has made me angry
73. P: Like this car accident.
74. C: Like this car accident.
75. P: Because it's so unfair.
76. C: Because it's so unfair.
77. P: It seems so unfair.
78. C: It seems so unfair.
79. P: And this car accident
80. C: And this car accident
81. P: Reminds me
82. C: Reminds me
83. P: That it's still unfair.
84. C: That it's still unfair.

Step 10 – Ask "Why would I put myself through this?"

85. P: Even though that happened as a child,
86. C: Even though that happened as a child,

87.   P: It is hard for me to imagine
88.   C: It is hard for me to imagine
89.   P: That I would ever put myself through such unfairness.
90.   C: That I would ever put myself through such unfairness.

Step 11 – Offer a valuable reason for choosing the event

91.   P: Yet nothing would exist unless it has value.
92.   C: Nothing would exist unless it has value.
93.   P: And this unfairness
94.   C: And this unfairness
95.   P: Is no exception.
96.   C: Is no exception.
97.   P: It absolutely has value.
98.   C: It absolutely has value.
99.   P: The display of unfairness
100.   C: The display of unfairness
101.   P: To me as a child
102.   C: To me as a child
103.   P: Has significant value
104.   C: Has significant value
105.   P: Because of that.
106.   C: Because of that.
107.   P: Because I was able to endure
108.   C: Because I was able to endure
109.   P: That unfairness
110.   C: That unfairness
111.   P: That anyone would call unfair.
112.   C: That anyone would call unfair.
113.   P: I grew by leaps and bounds.
114.   C: I grew by leaps and bounds.
115.   P: That's what I love most about myself.
116.   C: That's what I love most about myself.
117.   P: That I'm able to take that unfairness
118.   C: That I'm able to take that unfairness
119.   P: And continue my love.
120.   C: And continue my love.

121. P: It's been one of the hardest journeys of my life.
122. C: It's been one of the hardest journeys of my life.
123. P: But it's actually
124. C: But it's actually
125. P: What I love most about myself,
126. C: What I love most about myself,
127. P: My strength to love.
128. C: My strength to love.
129. P: Even during unfairness
130. C: Even during unfairness
131. P: I wanted that,
132. C: I wanted that,
133. P: Because I felt as though I was ready
134. C: Because I felt as though I was ready
135. P: To grow leaps and bounds
136. C: To grow leaps and bounds
137. P: Like a saint.
138. C: Like a saint.
139. P: It's been tough.
140. C: It's been tough.
141. P: I truly realize
142. C: I truly realize
143. P: Even now
144. C: Even now
145. P: That because
146. C: That because
147. P: I'm still able to love
148. C: I'm still able to love
149. P: Through the acts of unfairness,
150. C: Through the acts of unfairness,
151. P: It has made me love myself
152. C: It has made me love myself
153. P: Beyond my comprehension.
154. C: Beyond my comprehension.
155. P: I want to thank my sister

156. C: I want to thank my sister
157. P: For allowing me
158. C: For allowing me
159. P: The highest love for myself.
160. C: The highest love for myself.
161. P: I needed that.
162. C: I needed that.
163. P: Prior to that,
164. C: Prior to that,
165. P: I didn't love myself as much.
166. C: I didn't love myself as much.
167. P: Where I love myself
168. C: Where I love myself
169. P: A thousand times more now
170. C: A thousand times more now
171. P: Because of enduring that difficult time.
172. C: Because of enduring that difficult time.
173. P: This has been an amazing journey
174. C: This has been an amazing journey
175. P: Of self-love.
176. C: Of self-love.
177. P: So, this accident
178. C: So, this accident
179. P: That seemed unfair,
180. C: That seemed unfair,
181. P: That made me angry,
182. C: That made me angry,
183. P: Reminded me
184. C: Reminded me
185. P: That I was still
186. C: That I was still
187. P: Holding my sister prisoner,
188. C: Holding my sister prisoner,

Step 12 – Thank the childhood event and the people involved.

189. P: When in fact,

190. C: When in fact,
191. P: I should be thanking her
192. C: I should be thanking her
193. P: For helping me
194. C: For helping me
195. P: Love myself
196. C: Love myself
197. P: Beyond comprehension.
198. C: Beyond comprehension.
199. P: And I feel it in every bone in my body.
200. C: And I feel it in every bone in my body.
201. P: And it almost seems ridiculous.
202. C: And it almost seems ridiculous.
203. P: The act itself seems almost petty.
204. C: The act itself seems almost petty.
205. P: Yet I put so much on it
206. C: I put so much on it
207. P: Because so much was on it
208. C: Because so much was on it
209. P: Yet now I see it's petty.
210. C: Now I see it's petty.
211. P: And now I want to thank my sister
212. C: And now I want to thank my sister
213. P: For putting me through that difficult time.
214. C: For putting me through that difficult time.
215. P: I love myself beyond comprehension.
216. C: I love myself beyond comprehension.

Step 13 – Thank the original issue.

217. P: I want to thank the players of this accident
218. C: I want to thank the players of this accident
219. P: For giving me the opportunity
220. C: For giving me the opportunity
221. P: To free my sister,
222. C: To free my sister,
223. P: For how I've been keeping her in prison

224. C: For how I've been keeping her in prison
225. P: And allowing myself
226. C: And allowing myself
227. P: To recognize
228. C: To recognize
229. P: How much I've grown
230. C: How much I've grown
231. P: In loving myself.
232. C: In loving myself.

Step 14 – Stop tapping and get SUDS.

233. (Tapping stops)
234. P: How are you doing? On a scale to zero to ten
235. C: It's definitely come down. Like I don't feel anything in my chest anymore, so I feel it's not completely gone. I still feel anxious about driving. I don't trust some people around me.
236. P: So on a scale of zero to ten ...
237. C: Five.
238. P: Five, that's very, very good. Okay, where do you feel it now?
239. C: In my jaw.
240. P: In your jaw.
241. C: Very tense in my jaw.

(new issue) Step 2 – Get starting point issue (What, When, SUDS).

242. P: Very tense in your jaw. Okay. On scale from 0 to 10 where would you put that tenseness in your jaw?
243. C: A five.
244. P: A five, very, very good. Do you remember when you started to feel things in your jaw?
245. C: I tend to hold a lot of tension in my jaw.
246. P: Is there an emotion that might be with the tension in your jaw?
247. C: Anxiety and fear.
248. P: Ok, let's start tapping again.
249. (Tapping starts)

Step 4 – Begin Empathetic Bond.
Step 5 – Say what you know about the issue.

250. P: I'm holding this fear

251. C: I'm holding this fear
252. P: And anxiety in my jaw
253. C: And anxiety in my jaw

Step 6 – Make assumptions and repeat corrections.

254. P: Because that's what makes sense to me
255. C: Because that's what makes sense to me
256. P: And as I feel that in my jaw
257. C: And as I feel that in my jaw

Step 7 – Build client trust and learn about the issue.

258. P: It has a particular emotion to it.
259. C: It has a particular emotion to it.
260. P: It has a certain edge to it.
261. C: It has a certain edge to it.
262. P: As I focus on that discomfort in my jaw,
263. C: As I focus on that discomfort in my jaw,
264. P: I would like to say so what,
265. C: I would like to say so what,

Step 8 – Define the emotion.

266. P: But some emotion
267. C: But some emotion
268. P: Is preventing me from saying "so what."
269. C: Is preventing me from saying "so what."
270. P: Like I am bothered by something
271. C: Like I am bothered by something
272. P: Enough
273. C: Enough
274. P: To where I can't just say so what
275. C: To where I can't just say so what
276. P: And that emotion,
277. C: And that emotion,
278. P: That particular emotion,
279. C: That particular emotion,
280. P: Fear and anxiety
281. C: Fear and anxiety
282. P: And other emotions

283. C: And other emotions
284. P: Is familiar.
285. C: Is familiar.

Step 9 – Take the client back to the childhood event.

286. P: And like stepping through a window into the past
287. C: And like stepping through a window into the past
288. P: I can feel that sensation
289. C: I can feel that sensation
290. P: When I was a child
291. C: When I was a child
292. P: And how I kept it in my jaw
293. C: And how I kept it in my jaw
294. P: It's very familiar
295. C: It's very familiar
296. P: I remember the first time
297. C: I remember the first time
298. P: That I felt that, and I held that in my jaw.
299. C: That I felt that, and I held that in my jaw.
300. P: I held it in my jaw
301. C: I held it in my jaw
302. P: Because that's the only place I could keep it
303. C: Because that's the only place I could keep it
304. P: As a child,
305. C: As a child,
306. P: In my jaw.
307. C: In my jaw.
308. P: It's preventing myself to talk.
309. C: It's preventing myself to talk.
310. P: I'm holding that in my jaw
311. C: I'm holding that in my jaw
312. P: Because as a child
313. C: Because as a child
314. P: I could not speak my truth
315. C: I could not speak my truth. It was unsafe.
316. P: It was unsafe to speak my truth

317. C: It was unsafe to speak my truth
318. P: About my sister
319. C: About my sister
320. P: To someone else
321. C: To someone else
322. P: Or, to everyone. I remember where I was
323. C: I remember where I was
324. P: When I first held it tight in my jaw
325. C: When I first held it tight in my jaw
326. P: And I'm a very, very young girl.
327. C: I'm a very, very young girl.
328. P: But I held it tight in my jaw.
329. C: But I held it tight in my jaw.
330. P: Where am I? What's happening?
331. C: I see my backyard, but I don't see anyone around.
332. P: I see my backyard
333. C: I see my backyard
334. P: And all I know
335. C: And all I know
336. P: Is that
337. C: Is that
338. P: Somehow
339. C: Somehow
340. P: It doesn't matter
341. C: It doesn't matter
342. P: To other people
343. C: To other people
344. P: That I've been wronged,
345. C: That I've been wronged,
346. P: Clearly been wronged.
347. C: Clearly been wronged.
348. P: So, I have to hold it in my jaw.
349. C: So, I have to hold it in my jaw.
350. P: I've been shown
351. C: I've been shown

352. P: That I don't matter
353. C: That I don't matter
354. P: By the people in my backyard
355. C: By the people in my backyard
356. P: In that scene
357. C: In that scene
358. P: And I held it tight in my jaw.
359. C: And I held it tight in my jaw.
360. P: Maybe I walked out to the backyard by myself
361. C: Maybe I walked out to the backyard by myself
362. P: To get away from something.
363. C: To get away from something.
364. P: Something happened,
365. C: Something happened,
366. P: And I had to hold it in my jaw.
367. C: And I had to hold it in my jaw.
368. P: And I did.
369. C: And I did.
370. P: And it was hard.
371. C: And it was hard.
372. P: And that emotion
373. C: And that emotion
374. P: Is resentment.
375. C: Is resentment.

Step 10 – Ask "Why would I put myself through this?"

376. P: Why would I put myself through that?
377. C: Why would I put myself through that?
378. P: I did not have
379. C: I did not have
380. P: The rationalizing skills
381. C: The rationalizing skills
382. P: At that age
383. C: At that age
384. P: To be able just to say "so what."
385. C: To be able just to say "so what."

386. P: It's because I did not understand why
387. C: It's because I did not understand why
388. P: That that was happening.
389. C: That that was happening.
390. P: How could I be betrayed?
391. C: How could I be betrayed?
392. P: I cannot figure it out
393. C: I cannot figure it out
394. P: Because I don't have the rationalizing skills.
395. C: Because I don't have the rationalizing skills.
396. P: So, I put myself into a situation
397. C: So, I put myself into a situation
398. P: Where I had no coping skills
399. C: Where I had no coping skills
400. P: Because I'm so young.
401. C: Because I'm so young.
402. P: It is earlier than the age of eight.
403. C: It is earlier than the age of eight.
404. P: And I just don't understand why
405. C: And I just don't understand why
406. P: And even more so
407. C: And even more so
408. P: As a spirit.
409. C: As a spirit.
410. P: I don't know why I would put myself through that.
411. C: I don't know why I would put myself through that.
412. P: Yet nothing would exist
413. C: Yet nothing would exist
414. P: Unless it has value.
415. C: Unless it has value.
416. P: And putting me in that situation,
417. C: And putting me in that situation,
418. P: That unfair situation,
419. C: That unfair situation,
420. P: Where I don't understand

421. C: Where I don't understand
422. P: I don't understand why I was betrayed,
423. C: I don't understand why I was betrayed,
424. P: Why I have to keep my mouth shut,
425. C: Why I have to keep my mouth shut,
426. P: What am I ever going to learn from this.
427. C: What am I ever going to learn from this.
428. P: And as I look at that resentment
429. C: And as I look at that resentment
430. P: Now,
431. C: Now,
432. P: With my processing power
433. C: With my processing power
434. P: I can easily say "so what."
435. C: I can easily say "so what."
436. P: But that doesn't explain
437. C: But that doesn't explain
438. P: Why I was having such a tough time
439. C: Why I was having such a tough time
440. P: As a kid
441. C: As a kid
442. P: Because I didn't know
443. C: Because I didn't know
444. P: I now have to forgive.
445. C: I now have to forgive.
446. P: When I don't understand
447. C: When I don't understand
448. P: And that's why
449. C: And that's why
450. P: This situation exists,
451. C: This situation exists,
452. P: Because whoever it was
453. C: Because whoever it was
454. P: Was going through their own issues.
455. C: Was going through their own issues.

456. P: And now I realize,
457. C: And now I realize,
458. P: But back then I didn't.
459. C: But back then I didn't.

Step 11 – Offer a valuable reason for choosing the event

460. P: So, I've had to learn
461. C: So, I've had to learn
462. P: The extremely difficult task
463. C: The extremely difficult task
464. P: Of forgiving.
465. C: Of forgiving.
466. P: What I don't understand,
467. C: What I don't understand,
468. P: I have to forgive.
469. C: I have to forgive.
470. P: What I don't understand.
471. C: What I don't understand.
472. P: That is the greatest lesson of all.
473. C: That is the greatest lesson of all.
474. P: And I as I look back
475. C: And I as I look back
476. P: I see that I didn't understand,
477. C: I see that I didn't understand,
478. P: And yet now
479. C: And yet now
480. P: The fact that I've been able to still love
481. C: The fact that I've been able to still love
482. P: Even though I didn't understand
483. C: Even though I didn't understand
484. P: Has been one of the greatest accomplishments
485. C: Has been one of the greatest accomplishments
486. P: Of my lifetime.
487. C: Of my lifetime.
488. P: And what I love most about myself
489. C: And what I love most about myself

490. P: Is that I can forgive
491. C: Is that I can forgive
492. P: And I can love
493. C: And I can love
494. P: Even when I don't understand.
495. C: Even when I don't understand.
496. P: That was the whole purpose
497. C: That was the whole purpose
498. P: Of this difficult situation.
499. C: Of this difficult situation.
500. P: I see now where it was petty
501. C: I see now where it was petty
502. P: But back then I didn't.
503. C: But back then I didn't.
504. P: It was so emotionally trying for me.
505. C: It was so emotionally trying for me.
506. P: But now
507. C: But now
508. P: I look back and I see
509. C: I look back and I see
510. P: That my love has continued
511. C: That my love has continued
512. P: Even through these unfairnesses.
513. C: Even through these unfairnesses.
514. P: It has made me learn
515. C: It has made me learn
516. P: That I can
517. C: That I can
518. P: Forgive
519. C: Forgive
520. P: What I don't understand.
521. C: What I don't understand.
522. P: That's what I love most about myself.
523. C: That's what I love most about myself.
524. P: I feel it in my body.

525. C: I feel it in my body.
526. P: It has been really tough.
527. C: It has been really tough.
Step 12 – Thank the childhood event and the people involved.
528. P: I want to thank all the people in my lifetime
529. C: I want to thank all the people in my lifetime
530. P: For allowing me the opportunity
531. C: For allowing me the opportunity
532. P: To grow.
533. C: To grow.
534. P: For my love to grow.
535. C: For my love to grow.
536. P: To see
537. C: To see
538. P: That I can love
539. C: That I can love
540. P: Even though I don't understand.
541. C: Even though I don't understand.
542. P: I am a saint.
543. C: I am a saint.
544. P: It's been a tough, tough road
545. C: It's been a tough, tough road
546. P: But I'm ever so grateful.
547. C: But I'm ever so grateful.
548. P: I so want to thank them.
549. C: I so want to thank them.
550. P: I want to thank them when I was a child.
551. C: I want to thank them when I was a child.
552. P: My love is so big right now.
553. C: My love is so big right now.
554. P: It's a thousand times bigger
555. C: It's a thousand times bigger
556. P: Because of it.
557. C: Because of it.
Step 13 – Thank the original issue.

558. P: I want to thank again
559. C: I want to thank again
560. P: This seeming accident
561. C: This seeming accident
562. P: Has actually allowed me
563. C: Has actually allowed me
564. P: To look at myself
565. C: To look at myself
566. P: As I really have been:
567. C: As I really have been:
568. P: Someone who can love
569. C: Someone who can love
570. P: In the face of unfairness
571. C: In the face of unfairness
572. P: And when you don't understand
573. C: And when you don't understand

Step 14 – Stop tapping and get SUDS.
(2 rounds of silent tapping, then tapping stops.)
574. P: Upon a scale from zero to ten where would you put the discomfort in your jaw?
575. C: Zero.
576. P: Zero, on a scale of zero to ten where would you put the discomfort in your chest?
577. C: Zero.
578. P: God bless you.

Notes on Sample Session - C

This is a non-student client session where two or more issues typically come up in session. The PTSD from her car accident quickly identified more than one childhood traumatic experience of victimhood. This session demonstrates the power gained from self-responsibility and how an early-age difficult situation can heal PTSD.

Sample GEMT Session - C Follow-up Email from Client

This is the excerpt of the actual follow up email from the client in the session above three days after the GEMT session.

P: "It's been a few days since our session. How are things going?"
C: *"Thanks for checking in. I have to say that prior to our session, since the time of the accident, I had been unable to drive down the street where it took place because even the thought of it would cause me high anxiety and the start of panic attacks. This made getting to work very difficult and time consuming. Because of this, I went to see a therapist in hopes of getting help and relief from the anxiety. However, the therapist did not know how to help me. She was going to refer me to an EMDR specialist, but I had a GEMT session with you instead.*

The day after our session, for the first time since the accident, I drove to work down the street to the exact place the accident took place. I still had some feelings of anxiety start to come up when I was driving by for the first time, but I did it and I can't tell you how happy I am that I was able to! By the time I made the turn that I have been avoiding for about a month and a half, I was feeling no nervousness, no anxiety, no more feelings of panic. Thank you so much! This GEMT is amazing!"

Vocabulary of Feelings and Emotions

When working with a client who is having trouble identifying her emotions, you may want to offer some possibilities, so her subconscious has something to recognize. When a person hears the correct word that resonates within, there will be a response of recognition. Below are a few possible suggestions.

AFRAID
apprehensive	panic	foreboding	frightened
mistrust	terrified	petrified	scared

ANGRY
aggravated	dismayed	annoyed	displeased
frustrated	impatient	irritated	irked

CONFUSED
chaotic	baffled	bewildered	puzzled
hesitant	lost	stifled	perplexed

DISTURBED
unnerved	alarmed	disconcerted	uneasy
shocked	perturbed	rattled	restless

EMBARRASSED
ashamed	chagrined	flustered	guilty
mortified	self-conscious	humiliated	nervous

FATIGUED
beat	burnt-out	depleted	exhausted
lethargic	listless	worn-out	tired

HATE
animosity	appalled	contempt	disgust
repulsion	dislike	horrified	hostility

LONGING

envious	burning	yearning	nostalgic
pining	wanting	craving	aching

PAIN

agony	anguish	miserable	devastated
grief	heartbroken	hurt	lonely

REMOVED

alienated	numb	apathetic	disconnected
cold	detached	distant	distracted

SAD

depressed	dejected	despair	despondent
disappointed	discouraged	disheartened	hopeless

UPTIGHT

anxious	cranky	distressed	distraught
tense	frazzled	overwhelmed	stressed-out

VULNERABLE

fragile	guarded	helpless	insecure
leery	reserved	sensitive	shaky

Example of a GEMT Philosophy Dialogue

"I am the creator of my own experience? Really? I am not sure about that. If I am the creator of my own experience, then why would I create that particular situation? It sure looks like a mistake to me. Yet I cannot call it a mistake when I look at its positive aspects. When I look at how I benefited from that situation, I cannot call it a mistake. While I am focused on the positive aspects of anything, I cannot call it a mistake. In fact, the positive aspects of that situation are very particular. And all situations have particular positive aspects. I can only be a victim of a mistake, yet if there are no mistakes then I am never a victim. If I am never a victim, I must be the creator of my own experiences. Yet my experiences are the result of my choices, and this makes sense anyway. And, every choice I make, however silly, automatic, or quick, has positive aspects on some level else I would not make it. In fact, every decision I could possibly make has some positive aspect. In fact, everything has positive aspects. Is it that I am in resistance to seeing the positive aspects? Am I in resistance to seeing everything as growth? Am I in resistance to accepting what is? Am I trying to fix or change the past instead of changing my perception about it? Am I in resistance to seeing the perfection of what is? How am I going to help my clients with GEMT if I cannot see their situation as the perfect manifestation of their choices with many particular positive aspects? How am I going to see them as creators of their own experience, when I am in resistance to seeing myself as creator of my own experience? I am the creator of my own experience? Really?"

Quiz Answers

Quiz Answers Part 1

1) Why is "Meridian Tapping" used as part of the modality name rather than "desensitization" or "emotional anesthesia"?
   a) Incorrect: Part 1 – The GEMT Method: GEMT is not similar to other tapping modalities because it does not focus on fixing, modifying, or removing symptoms, seeing them as an effect, not a cause.
   b) Incorrect: Part 1 – The GEMT Method: Meridian tapping itself does not do the healing, but it provides what we call a temporary "emotional anesthesia" which reduces negative emotions and defensiveness about the ailment, so that practitioners can empathetically guide clients to a perspective that their ailment has value.
   c) CORRECT: Intro: This level of healing would be nearly impossible without both emotional anesthesia and empathetic rapport, and the reason why meridian tapping is in the name of this modality.
   d) Incorrect: Part 1 – What is Healing?: Unlike some modalities, you need not be a licensed acupuncturist or mental health professional to be a GEMT practitioner.

2) GEMT differs from other modalities because
   a) True: Part 1 – The GEMT Method: One of the unique qualities that makes GEMT different from other modalities is that it does not focus on healing the dis-ease; it focuses on healing the reaction to the dis-ease, and when the reaction is healed (understood, transformed, transmuted) there no longer seems to be a need or use for the dis-ease.
   b) True: Part 1 - GEMT Compared to EFT: GEMT differs from EFT in that the client and practitioner will thank the ailment and the people involved for bringing the opportunity for healing a difficult event from the past.

c) True: Part 1 - The Problem GEMT Solves: GEMT views past events as perfect and brilliant creations of the client and is one of the ways it differs from other modalities.

d) CORRECT: All the above

3) How does GEMT view disease?
   a) True: Part 1 – What is Disease?: Regardless of the ailment and for the purpose of a GEMT session, we simply say, "disease is an effect of misperception."
   b) True: Part 1 – What is Disease?: In GEMT, manifested disease is cherished for its emotional aspects which are the key indicators to finding the core misperception.
   c) True: Part 1 – What is Disease?: Beyond that, defining, analyzing or focusing on the facets or discord of a disease is unnecessary, and may have the adverse effect of giving it deeper roots.
   d) CORRECT: All the above.

Quiz Answers Part 2

1) What type of people are we influenced by most?
   a) Incorrect: Part 2 – Empathetic Influence: We are occasionally influenced by experts, successful people, and people we like and admire, but we are most influenced by the people who understand us.
   b) Incorrect: Part 2 – Empathetic Influence: We are occasionally influenced by experts, successful people, and people we like and admire, but we are most influenced by the people who understand us.
   c) CORRECT: Part 2 – Empathetic Influence: We are occasionally influenced by experts, successful people, and people we like and admire, but we are most influenced by the people who understand us.
   d) Incorrect: Part 2 – Empathetic Influence: We are occasionally influenced by experts, successful people, and people we like

and admire, but we are most influenced by the people who understand us.

2) You realize you feel emotionally neutral about a client's situation or disease. What can you do to minimize the risk of harming the client?
   a) Incorrect: Part 2 – Do No Harm: If your feelings are neutral about the client's situation, you are actually in resistance to it being "good" or a beneficial presence, an indication that there must be something about their unchangeable past with which you don't agree.
   b) CORRECT: Part 2 – Do No Harm: When you realize you feel emotionally neutral about a client's situation or disease, take the stance that there must be a major upside, but it is currently beyond comprehension.
   c) Incorrect: Part 2 – How to Perceive the Client: Coddling a client with extra kindness can be harmful because it risks her thinking that you think she is helpless, weak or a victim, or that her manifestation is bad.
   d) Incorrect: Part 2 – Empathy vs. Sympathy: Empathy can heal with its understanding, but sympathy could be considered harmful when it perceives or judges a situation as bad.

3) What have desensitization techniques brought to cognitive healing modalities?
   a) CORRECT: Part 2 – Desensitization Therapies and Meridian Tapping: All desensitization therapies have proven to give temporary relief of fears, phobias and painful memories so they can be confronted with minimal discomfort.
   b) Incorrect: Part 2 – Desensitization Therapies and Meridian Tapping: Our experiences disallow us from concurring with the claims that desensitization therapies alone can permanently remove negative emotions, cure diseases, and even forgive by tapping on forgiveness meridian points (pinky and index fingers).

c) Incorrect: Part 2 – Desensitization Therapies and Meridian Tapping: Our experiences disallow us from concurring with the claims that desensitization therapies alone can permanently remove negative emotions, cure diseases, and even forgive by tapping on forgiveness meridian points (pinky and index fingers).

d) Incorrect: Part2 – Desensitization Therapies and Meridian Tapping: Our experiences disallow us from concurring with the claims that desensitization therapies alone can permanently remove negative emotions, cure diseases, and even forgive by tapping on forgiveness meridian points (pinky and index fingers).

4) Your client is overreacting while sharing a story about an interaction with another person. What is your best response?

   a) Incorrect: Part 2 – The Healing Power of Empathy: Often, when someone overreacts and turns to us for comfort, we unconsciously dismiss her reaction and share our elevated perspective about the situation, which can add to her dis-ease.

   b) Incorrect: Part 2 – The Healing Power of Empathy: If we fall into the trap of trying to "teach" her to see it our way or set aside her feelings and empathize with those she believes have hurt her, we invalidate her and her feelings.

   c) Incorrect: Part 2 – The Healing Power of Empathy: This is the time to empathize and not the best time to advise, mediate, problem-solve, or remind her there are many ways to perceive a situation.

   d) CORRECT: Part 2 – Emotional Agreement: The highest level of empathetic healing is to fully validate the client by completely agreeing with her response and feelings about the situation.

5) Which is the most ideal way to perceive a client?

   a) Incorrect: Part 2 – How to Perceive the Client: If the client is viewed as someone who needs your help to solve her problems or who has an ailment you are confident you can remove; the session is now less about what is best for the client and more about validating you as a successful healer.

b) CORRECT: Part 2 – How to Perceive the Client: The most ideal way to perceive your client is that she is part of you and everything that exists.

c) Incorrect: Part 2 – How to Perceive the Client: If the client is viewed as someone who needs your help to solve her problems or who has an ailment you are confident you can remove; the session is now less about what is best for the client and more about validating you as a successful healer.

d) Incorrect: Part 2 – How to Perceive the Client: New practitioners who develop this unconscious perspective of viewing a client as another person who will validate how great a healer they are often wonder why their client base is low.

Quiz Answers Part 3

1) Excellent GEMT practitioners are

a) CORRECT: Part 3 – Courage and the Practitioner: Almost anyone who believes with certainty that nothing would exist unless it had value can be an excellent GEMT practitioner.

b) Incorrect: Part 3 – Courage and the Practitioner: The concepts of forgiveness work, though they may be useful in other contexts, still portray the client as a victim.

c) Incorrect: Part 3 – Courage and the Practitioner: GEMT attempts to start the session as quickly as possible rather than having the client talk through her issues.

d) Incorrect: Part 3 – Courage and the Practitioner: Many analysts are brilliant in their problem-solving skills; however, in GEMT there are no problems to solve.

2) You have just facilitated a GEMT session where the client ultimately resolved her chronic pain which has kept her in a

wheelchair for years. While in a department store, you see a man in a wheelchair and, feeling confident from the session earlier, have the urge to approach him to offer your help healing his ailment. How would this be inappropriate and potentially harmful to him?

a) Incorrect: Part 2 – Want What is Best for Your Client: "Wants" of the practitioner create expectations for the client, and these expectations can be a precursor to judgment.

b) Incorrect: Part 3 – The Purpose of a GEMT Practitioner: It is also important to be aware that a practitioner's attention can have the adverse effect of prolonging or worsening the victim mentality or self-destructive behavior of those not ready to heal when the purpose of their dis-ease is to attract attention.

c) Incorrect: Part 3 – The Purpose of a GEMT Practitioner: There are some who do not perceive themselves as victims because they are experiencing benefits from their ailment and any offer to help them would be introducing judgment.

d) CORRECT: All the above

3) You have a new client who wants to see you for arthritis, which reminds you of your aunt's painful bout with the disease. What is best to do before the session?

a) Incorrect: Part 3 – When to Refer a Client: Instead of immediately referring to a client who has an ailment you have a negative association with, attempt to have an imaginary session where the ailment is viewed as a perfect metaphor to change a negative perspective.

b) CORRECT: Part 3 – When to Refer a Client: Instead of immediately referring to a client who has an ailment you have a negative association with, attempt to have an imaginary session where the ailment is viewed as a perfect metaphor to change a negative perspective.

c) Incorrect: Part 3 – Medical Knowledge: In GEMT all physical ailments are converted into emotional discomforts, so knowledge beyond a basic understanding of the ailment is not necessary.

d) Incorrect: Part 3 – Discussions with New or Potential Clients: When a practitioner shares sympathetic personal stories of struggles with ailments, it risks increasing dis-ease as well as takes the focus away from the client.

4) A new client calls to make an appointment with you for a chronic disease she feels that she has had since birth. Because symptoms seem to come and go at random, she feels the ailment is controlling her life. While on the phone with her, what aspects of the session should you discuss?
   a) Incorrect: Part 3 – Discussions with New or Potential Clients: Either way, we avoid talking about past lives and karma prior to a session.
   b) Incorrect: Part 3 – Discussions with New or Potential Clients: There exists a potentially volatile situation prior to a session such that any mention of them being the creator of their illness or discomfort could cause significant resistance and adverse reactions.
   c) CORRECT: Part 3 – Discussions with new or potential clients: It is always a good idea to remind the client to not use drugs or alcohol prior to a session.
   d) Incorrect: All the above.

5) Which questions are helpful when not in an empathetic bond?
   a) Incorrect: Part 3 – Questions and Statements When Not in Empathetic Bond: Even a seemingly helpful question like "What would you like to have happen?" would invariably solicit a response to remove, fix, or modify a symptom and bypass why it might be valuable.
   b) Incorrect: Part 3 – Questions and Statements When Not in Empathetic Bond: It is also important to refrain from asking closed, interrogative or combative questions such as "What is the value of your ailment?" or "How is your ailment serving you?"

c) CORRECT: Part 3 – Questions and Statements When Not in Empathetic Bond: Answers to questions such as "What feelings are coming up?" and "What situations are you remembering?" are key to finding the core issue.

d) Incorrect: All the above

Quiz Answers Part 4

1) You have identified the ailment, established SUDS and are about to start the session, but the client feels like she has not talked enough about her issue or you have not asked enough questions. What is the best way to handle this situation?

   a) Incorrect: Part 4 – Note-taking with GEMT: Because the original issue is viewed as an alert to look at something bigger, in-depth interview questions or notes are not needed or recommended because it is not the focus of the session.

   b) Incorrect: Part 4 – GEMT Session Conversation: It is important to not assume in any way that you know what the issue is or where the conversation is going to go.

   c) Incorrect: Part 4 – Start Tapping: Delaying the tapping to talk more about the issue can lower the client's vibration and even cause the starting point issue to change.

   d) CORRECT: Part 4 – Start Tapping: If the client wants to talk more about her issue at this time, explain that it is best to begin tapping while continuing the conversation and see where things go.

2) The client has repeated the starting point details in Empathetic Bond. However, as you start to lead with assumptions, the client stops repeating. What should you do first?

   a) Incorrect: Part 4 – Contrasting Thoughts: Pausing the session when the client is not repeating risks losing rapport and should only be done if you feel confident that a question like "What is coming up?" will have an answer.

b) Incorrect: Part 4 – Stalling: Avoid stalling when the client is not repeating because it risks losing rapport and might be perceived as belittling.

c) CORRECT: Part 4 – Contrasting Thoughts: The best option when a client is not repeating is to first offer contrasting thoughts.

d) Incorrect: Part 4 –What if the Client Stops Repeating?: If the client stops repeating while in an empathetic bond, try contrasting thoughts instead of repeating the statement or going down a different path.

3) While leading your client, you make an erroneous assumption about her ailment and she corrects you. What is the best course of action?

a) Incorrect: Part 4 – GEMT Session Conversation: Incorrect assumptions are inevitable and even deliberate at times, so there is never a need to apologize.

b) CORRECT: Part 4 – GEMT Session Conversation: It is, however, important for the practitioner to repeat verbatim the client's corrections with "I" statements to maintain the empathetic bond and increase rapport.

c) Incorrect: Part 4 – GEMT Session Conversation: It is, however, important for the practitioner to repeat verbatim the client's corrections with "I" statements to maintain the empathetic bond and increase rapport.

d) Incorrect: Part 4 – GEMT Session Conversation: Pausing the session during a correction risks losing rapport.

4) You have identified the emotion associated with the current ailment but then you become stuck, not knowing where to go next. What is ideal?

a) CORRECT: Part 4 – GEMT Session Conversation: GEMT basic flow outline: Uncover a childhood traumatic event with a similar emotion.

b) Incorrect: Part 4 – GEMT Session Conversation: It is not ideal for the client to suspect you are stuck by you awkwardly pausing the session or for you to verbally disclose it to her.

c) Incorrect: Part 4 – GEMT Session Conversation: GEMT basic flow outline: Once converted, physical aspects will not be discussed until the end of the session.

d) Incorrect: Part 4 – GEMT Session Conversation: It is not ideal for the client to suspect you are stuck by you awkwardly pausing the session or for you to verbally disclose it to her.

5) Just minutes after starting the session the client is surprised and overwhelmed as she begins remembering a childhood traumatic event she has not thought about in decades. What is the best course of action?

a) Incorrect: Part 4 – Reading the Nuances of Client Feedback: Important points to remember when a client is overwhelmed: Stay in an empathetic bond with "I" statements and do not make or imply "you" questions or statements.

b) Incorrect: Part 4 – Reading the Nuances of Client Feedback: Important points to remember when a client is overwhelmed: Continue tapping and do not pause the session. Encourage the client to begin tapping again if she has stopped.

c) Incorrect: Part 4 – Reading the Nuances of Client Feedback: Important points to remember when a client is overwhelmed: Lead with powerful affirmations and stop giving attention to the event.

d) CORRECT: Part 4 – Reading the Nuances of Client Feedback: Important points to remember when a client is overwhelmed: Stall by continuing to tap, slowing down words and breaking up sentences. Add more emotional anesthesia (side-to-side eye movement, deep breathing).

6) Your client has just fully confronted her childhood core issue while you empathetically validated her feelings and actions. What is the

most important statement to make while in an empathetic bond at this time?

   a) Incorrect: Part 4 – Planting the Seed of Responsibility: Once the core issue is found, for the remainder of the session there is no blaming, assigning of fault, or even forgiveness.
   b) Incorrect: Part 4 – Planting the Seed of Responsibility: Once the core issue is found, for the remainder of the session there is no blaming, assigning of fault, or even forgiveness.
   c) CORRECT: Part 4 – Planting the Seed of Responsibility: Here are example statements of planting the seed of responsibility: "Why would I put myself through this?"
   d) Incorrect: Part 4 – Planting the Seed of Responsibility: Once the core issue is found, for the remainder of the session there is no blaming, assigning of fault, or even forgiveness.

7) In Empathetic Bond, you are intuitively guided to suggest that the enormous value of her childhood traumatic event was to be free of a subconscious guilt that has plagued her for lifetimes. This being the apex of the session, you leverage your empathetic influence and give enormous value to the childhood traumatic event for her to take responsibility for it. What is the ultimate reason for this?

   a) CORRECT: Part 1 – What is GEMT?: The ultimate goal of GEMT is to facilitate the client's understanding that she is not a victim and is responsible for manifesting her ailment so that she can choose to heal it.
   b) Incorrect: Part 1 – The GEMT Method: GEMT is not similar to other tapping modalities because it does not focus on fixing, modifying, or removing symptoms, seeing them as an effect, not a cause.
   c) Incorrect: Part 1 – Beneficial Side Effects: At certain times we all innocently play healing roles for each other… However, this is not the reason or the focus of the GEMT session.
   d) Incorrect: Part 1 – Beneficial Side Effects: Everything has value; suffering and dis-ease are no exceptions… However, this is not the reason or the focus of the GEMT session.

References

A Course in Miracles, Helen Schucman
Ask and It Is Given, Esther Hicks
Eye Movement Desensitization and Reprocessing (EMDR) Therapy,
Francine Shapiro
How To Win Friends and Influence People, Dale Carnegie
Hypnosis and Hypnotherapy, Calvin D. Banyan
Hypnosis for Change, Josie Hadley and Carol Staudacher
Men Are from Mars, Women Are from Venus, John Gray
Mind Over Medicine, Lisa Rankin, MD
Molecules of Emotion, Candice Pert, PhD
My Method, Émile Coué
Neuro-linguistic Programming, Volume I, Dilts, Grinder, Bandler,
DeLozier
Nonviolent Communication, Marshall B. Rosenberg
Power vs. Force, David R. Hawkins M.D. PhD.
Professional Hypnotism Manual, John G. Kappas, PhD
Reinventing Medicine, Larry Dossey, MD
Self Mastery Through Conscious Autosuggestion, Émile Coué
The 5 Love Languages, Gary Chapman
The Biology of Belief, Bruce Lipton, PhD
The Biology of Perception, The Psychology of Change (DVD), Bruce
Lipton, PhD
The Divine Matrix, Gregg Braden
The EFT Manual, Gary Craig
The I Am Discourses, Volume 3, Guy W. Ballard
The Kybalion, Three Initiates
The Law of One (AKA: The Ra Material), Don Elkins
The Miracle Within, Émile Coué
The Power of Now, Eckhart Tolle
The Quimby Manuscripts, Phineas Parkhurst Quimby
The Wisdom of Your Cells: How Your Beliefs Control Your Biology,
Bruce Lipton, PhD
The Work of The Digestive Glands, Ivan Pavlov
This School Called Planet Earth, Summer Bacon

GEMT Practice Session Worksheet

Three things I know:
1. The client is the creator and never a victim.
2. The issue is a re-stimulation of an event prior to reasoning skills.
3. Nothing would exist unless it had value.

① Say client's name and raise vibration

② Get starting point issue (What, When, SUDS)

③ Start tapping while explaining the process

④ Begin Empathetic Bond "So, I have this __"

⑤ Say what you know (What, When, SUDS)

⑥ Make assumptions and repeat corrections

⑦ Build client's trust while learning about the issue

⑧ Define the emotion about the issue

⑨ Take client back to similar emotion in childhood

⑩ Ask "Why would I put myself through this?"

⑪ Offer a valuable reason for choosing the event

⑫ Thank the event and the people for the value

⑬ Thank original issue for the opportunity to heal

⑭ Stop tapping, get the starting point issue SUDS

⑮ Anchor healing with hypnotherapy